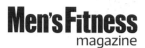

THE ULTIMATE GUIDE TO
FAT LOSS

by Joe Warner

Art Editor Fanni Williams

Chief Sub Editor Jo Williams

Art Director Donovan Walker

Photography Duncan Nicholls, Shutterstock

Model Oliver Jedrej@WAthletic

Cover model David Lancaster@WAthletic

Illustrations Sudden Impact

With thanks to Ultimate Performance (upfitness.co.uk)

MAGBOOK

Group Publisher **Russell Blackman**
Group Managing Director **Ian Westwood**
International Business Development Director
Dharmesh Mistry
Digital Production Manager **Nicky Baker**
Operations Director **Robin Ryan**
Managing Director of Advertising
Julian Lloyd-Evans
Newstrade Director **David Barker**
Managing Director of Enterprise **Martin Belson**
Chief Operating Officer/
Chief Financial Officer **Brett Reynolds**
Group Finance Director **Ian Leggett**
Chief Executive Officer **James Tye**
Chairman **Felix Dennis**

The 'MagBook' brand is a trademark of Dennis Publishing Ltd,
30 Cleveland Street, London W1T 4JD.
Company registered in England.
All material © Dennis Publishing Ltd, licensed by Felden 2013,
and may not be reproduced in whole or part without the
consent of the publishers. Printed at Polestar Bicester.

THE ULTIMATE GUIDE TO FAT LOSS ISBN **1-78106-139-4**
To license this product please contact Nicole Adams on
+44 (0) 20 7907 6134 or nicole_adams@dennis.co.uk

Advertising
Katie Wood katie_wood@dennis.co.uk
Emma D'Arcy emma_darcy@dennis.co.uk

To subscribe to *Men's Fitness* magazine,
call **0844 844 0081** or go to **mensfitness.co.uk**

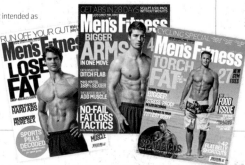

CONTENTS

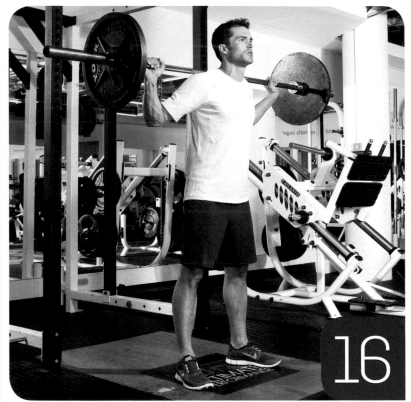

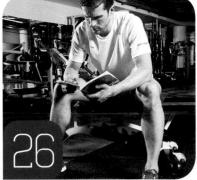

26

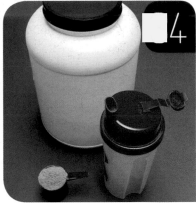

4

16

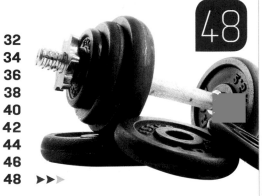

48

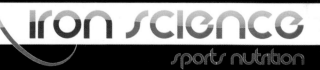

CONTENTS

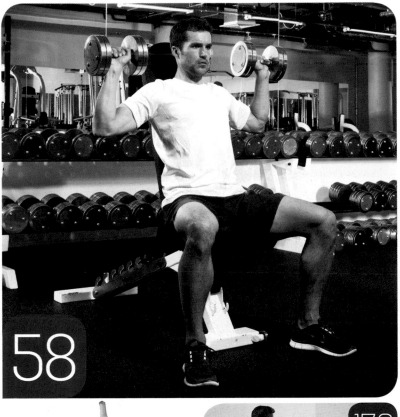

58

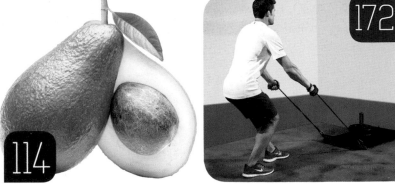

172

114

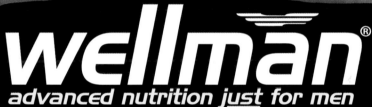
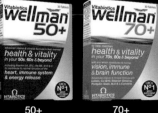

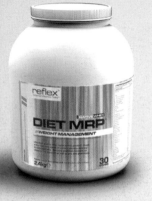

IT'S ALL IN THE
NUMBERS

44.8^g
Carbohydrate

175^{mg}
Magnesium

37.5^{mg}
Vitamin C

31^{µg}
Vitamin K2 MK-7

6.2^{µg}
Vitamin D3

7.5^{mg}
Vitamin E
(DeltaGold®)

40^g
Protein

per 100g

Eating a healthy calorie controlled and balanced diet whilst living a modern lifestyle is not always possible. Diet MRP® replaces a complete meal and provides a guaranteed balance of protein, carbohydrate and fat in conjunction with a broad spectrum of vitamins, minerals and antioxidants.

It contains low glycemic index carbohydrate sources; oats, barley and trehalose. Lower GI sources of carbohydrates are broken down slowly, providing energy over a longer period of time, allowing for a more balanced release of energy than simple carbohydrate sources such as dextrose or sucrose which are used extensively in many cheaper meal replacements. Additionally, oats and barley are rich in other nutrients such as fibre and naturally occurring vitamins and minerals.

Diet MRP® contains a unique multivitamin and mineral complex which is simply not found in other meal replacements. Each serving of Diet MRP® contains high quality amino acid chelated minerals; there are no cheap oxide forms of minerals like magnesium oxide or zinc oxide. You will also find the very rare form of vitamin E called DeltaGold® delta-tocotrienol and MenaquineGold™ vitamin K2 MK7. A full vitamin B complex is also present, with the addition of LactoSpore® pro-biotics.

£39.99
@ www.reflex-nutrition.com

 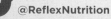

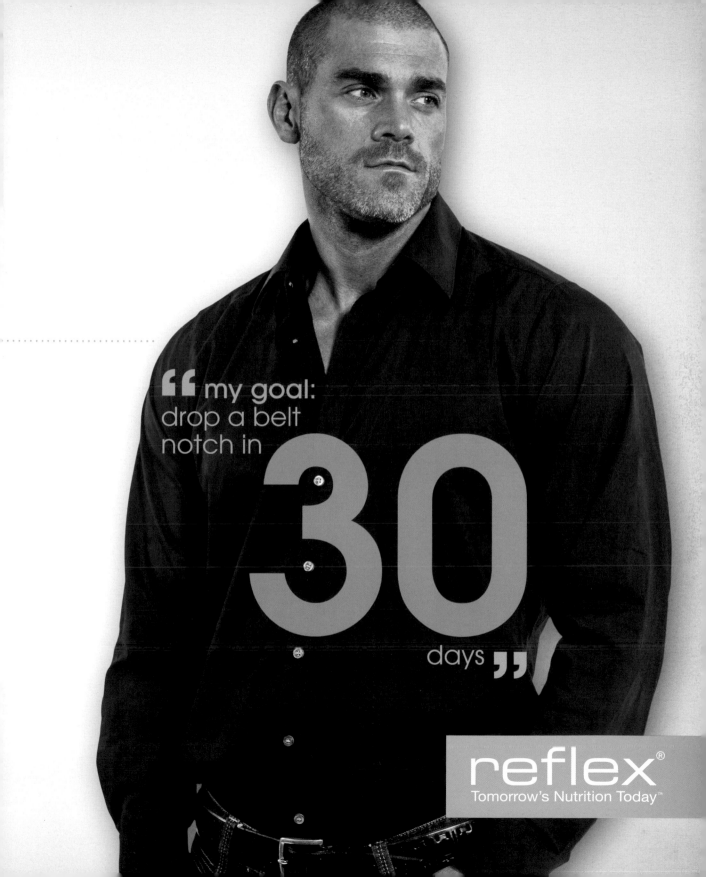

ABOUT THE BOOK

Welcome to the only guide to burning fat that you'll ever need

There are many reasons for wanting to lose weight. Maybe you have a beach holiday coming up and want to look better with your top off. Or perhaps you're getting married and want to make sure your morning suit fits in all the right places. Or maybe you just want to become fitter and healthier to get more out of your life.

Whatever your reason for wanting to getting rid of any excess body fat, you've come to the right place. This book is your definitive guide to getting into better shape, and the beauty of it is that you can transform your body in just six weeks.

Everything you need to know is clearly explained over the following pages. The first chapter details the fundamental principles behind burning body fat, both from an exercise and nutrition perspective, and contains a comprehensive overview of how this book's six-week training and diet plan works so you can follow it to the letter to get the best results possible.

There's also an in-depth guide to the supplements you can take to enhance your effort, so you get even better results more quickly, as well as answers to some of your most common fitness, health and nutrition questions.

After that we get straight into the six-week training and diet programme, which has been designed to burn away body fat while also adding lean muscle mass to completely transform your physique. How this programme works is explained fully on p14.

So whatever your motivation for taking positive steps to lose weight, your six-week journey to a better, leaner and healthier body starts here. What are you waiting for?

Joe Warner
Editor

ABOUT THE AUTHOR

Joe Warner is a journalist and author specialising in health and fitness. He's the co-author of *12-Week Body Plan*, the Amazon.co.uk best-selling book detailing the workouts and diet he followed to transform his physique from that of an out-of-shape journalist into the cover model of the September 2012 issue of *Men's Fitness* magazine. He has also written the *Total Training Guide* – which contains every exercise you'll ever need to build muscle and burn fat – and the forthcoming *Build Rock-Hard Abs*. All these MagBooks are available from Amazon.co.uk.

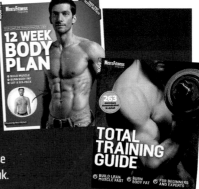

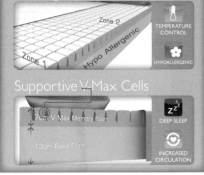
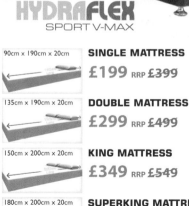

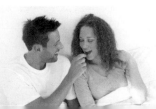

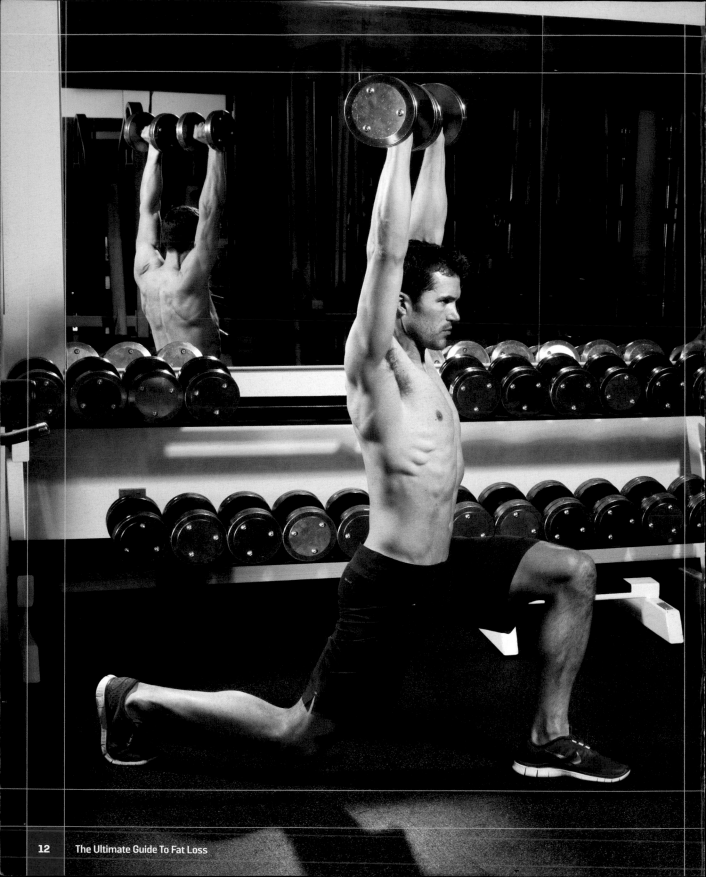

INTRODUCTION

Read this chapter to discover how
you will transform your physique
over the next six weeks

SIX WEEKS TO A NEW YOU

You're less than two months away from a leaner, healthier body

Building a leaner, fitter and healthier body is simple as long as you exercise correctly and eat the right foods at the right times. That's why this book is different from many other fat-loss guides. In it you'll find detailed guides to the workouts you need to complete and what you need to eat and why.

The six-week programme has been broken into weekly chapters that not only tell you when and how to train, but also contain a meal plan so you know what to eat to give you the best possible chance of building a better body.

CHAPTER BREAKDOWN

Each of the six weekly chapters in this book follows the same pattern. It starts with an introduction to that week's training and nutrition plan, followed by a two-page meal plan telling you what to eat over those seven days. Then come the training sessions you need to complete in order, including detailed form guides to ensure you perform each exercise correctly.

This programme requires you to complete four workouts each week: three weight-training

You won't find any long cardio sessions in this plan because steady-state cardio is an ineffective way to burn fat

sessions and one short, intense cardio workout. You won't find any long cardio sessions in this plan because steady-state cardio is an ineffective way to burn fat, especially when compared with weight training and high-intensity cardio (see Training For Fat Loss, p16, for further details).

Each of the three weight-based workouts each week concentrates on a different part of the body: the first is an upper-body session, the second works the lower body and the third is a total-body workout.

TRAINING SECRETS

Training multiple muscle groups in the same workout is one of the most effective ways to get your heart rate high and create an oxygen debt. Both of these fire up your metabolism – the rate at which your body burns calories – and mobilise your fat stores to be burned as energy.

At the end of each of the three weekly workouts you'll see a suggested Fat-Loss Finisher – a move designed to push your body even further out of its

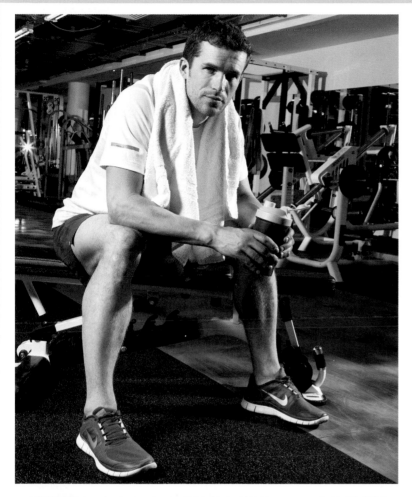

comfort zone so you burn even more fat (see p172 for details).

The fourth and final workout each week is a high-intensity cardio session. This complements the work you've already done in the weights room to blast away body fat and improve your cardiovascular fitness – how efficiently your heart and lungs work together to pump blood, oxygen and other essential nutrients around your body.

It also has the additional benefit of releasing more of the hormones that burn fat and build muscle, as well as making you fitter so you can push yourself harder in the gym.

BRAND NEW YOU

All you need to do is stick to the seven-day meal plans and perform the four weekly sessions in order and you'll start shedding body fat at a rate that until now you thought impossible, giving you a brand new body in just six weeks.

MAKE THE MOST OF IT

Follow these tips to make this six-week fat-loss programme work for you

Gain a solid understanding of how to train and eat to burn fat. Start with our in-depth look at the best training techniques for fat loss (p16) and which foods are best when it comes to reducing body fat (p20). You'll also find an explanation of how your body builds muscle (p42) and how to mobilise your stores of body fat to be burned as energy (p44).

It's important you follow the weekly training plans. Turn to p24 for an explanation of how each workout is put together and how you should perform it, plus a list of all the workout sessions you'll complete over the six weeks.

Turn to p30 to see how the nutrition plans work so you can follow the eating plan perfectly for the best results.

For the latest research on which supplements you may consider taking to accelerate your fat-burning and muscle-building mission, turn to p34.

Still got questions? We've got the answers to common queries about training (p28), diet (p32) and fitness (p46), as well as a glossary of common fitness terms (p48).

TRAINING FOR FAT LOSS

Discover the best way to exercise if you want to burn fat

Your body wants you to be fat. Not obese or overweight, but not so lean that your six-pack is on show either. It isn't that it's incredibly modest, but from an evolutionary perspective excess body fat is what kept your ancestors alive. When food was scarce their fat stores gave them the energy to survive and, more importantly, breed. It's how you're here today, reading this book.

But just because your body wants to maintain a decent level of body fat to ensure your survival should times turn tough, it doesn't mean you can't significantly reduce the amount you carry by following the right training and nutrition plan.

DO IT RIGHT
However, if you thought the best way to burn away your excess body fat was to go for regular

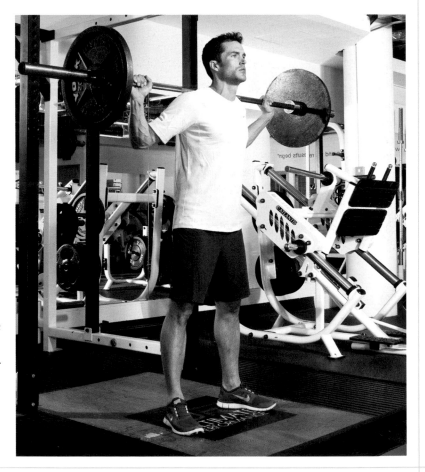

long-distance runs at a steady pace, it's time to think again.

For years people have mistakenly believed steady-state cardio endurance exercise is the most effective method to lose weight. In fact, regularly performing such long, slow sessions – whether of running, rowing, cycling or swimming – isn't the right way to get thinner. This is especially true if such training is complemented by a nutrition plan based around carbohydrates such as pasta, potatoes and bread.

OPPOSITE EFFECT

In some cases too much cardio training can actually lead to an increase in body fat because running for hours on end places a great deal of stress on your body. An increase in the stress hormone cortisol instructs your body to store more of the energy you consume as fat and also has a nasty side effect of breaking down muscle tissue.

Long, slow sessions do not keep your body into the mythical 'fat-burning zone', where body fat is prioritised over other energy stores to fuel your efforts (see the box, below). Still need convincing? Just look at amateur marathon runners. The majority don't have rippling muscles, lean waists or six-packs.

GET INTENSE

The best method of torching body fat is to combine weight training with high-Intensity cardio sessions, during which you run, row or cycle at intense levels for short periods.

Both these methods have a similar effect on your body. They cause a spike in testosterone – the male sex hormone responsible for a host of functions ranging

from increased libido to higher muscle and lower body-fat levels. Levels of human growth hormone are also heightened after weight-training workouts, which instructs your body to burn fat and build new muscle tissue.

Weight training and high-intensity cardio also significantly work your cardiovascular system. Increasing the rate at which your heart and lungs have tu work to pump blood, oxygen and other

> ❝ The best method of torching body fat is to combine weight training with high-intensity sessions of running, rowing or cycling ❞

nutrients around your body has a positive effect on reducing body-fat levels.

DEBT PAID

During intense periods of exercise your lungs can't take in enough oxygen to provide your ▶▶▶

TAKEAWAY TIPS

Key points to remember when training for fat loss

KEEP THE PACE

You need to work hard and fast, so stick to the tempo and rest periods detailed in each workout table. If you are able to talk while training, you're not working hard enough.

DON'T GET COMFORTABLE

If you find a session too easy, you need to make it harder. If you're sticking to the required sets, reps, tempo and rest periods and are still coasting, increase the weight you're lifting. You need to give your all at every single session.

STAY ACTIVE

A sedentary, deskbound lifestyle is one of the biggest causes of weight gain. The more you can get out and about during your everyday life, the better your chances of success. This may be as simple as taking stairs at work or walking to meetings instead of getting a taxi. The more you move, the more you prime your body to burn fat.

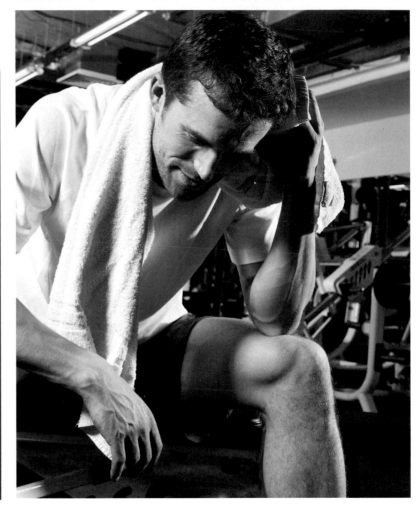

body with what it needs. This has the effect of creating an 'oxygen debt' within your body.

Just like any debt, this deficit needs to be repaid. Your body does this by increasing the amount of oxygen it consumes in the hours after your exercise session has finished. This phenomenon is known as excess post-exercise oxygen consumption, or EPOC,

❝Simply picking up a heavy bar once and then walking away isn't the right approach to take❞

and this period of increased oxygen intake also increases the rate at which you burn calories (for a more detailed

explanation of how EPOC works to burn fat, see the box, right).

Another benefit of any form of high-intensity exercise is that it causes lactic acid to accumulate in your muscle cells. While this build-up is responsible for the unpleasant feelings of 'muscle burn', elevated levels of this compound – which is a by-product of glucose metabolism – are thought to lead to an increase in the release of fat-torching growth hormones in the hours following your workout.

REST ASSURED
But while lifting weights is one of the best ways to burn fat, simply picking up a heavy bar once and then walking away isn't the right approach to take. Yes, doing so will eventually make you stronger, but it will have very little effect on your body fat levels.

You need to lift weights in a specific way to elicit the desired fat-burning response. For this programme that means you need to approach your three weekly weight training sessions in the same manner as you do the cardio session. That means working hard for a set period and then taking a short rest before lifting again.

Never giving your body quite enough time to recover is critical to whether your efforts to burn fat will be successful or not. This technique, which really pushes you out of your comfort zone, is known as 'accumulated fatigue' and results in the maximum number of muscle fibres being broken down. It's also responsible for elevating lactic acids in your muscles and forcing your heart and lungs to work really hard. These factors combine to increase lean muscle mass and reduce fat stores to give you a better body.

> ❝ Never giving your body quite enough time to recover is critical to whether your efforts to burn fat will be successful ❞

That's why the workouts in this book are based around two giant sets of four moves. Taking very little rest between each individual exercise keeps your heart rate high and does the maximum amount of damage to your muscles, so it's vital you stick rigidly to the rest periods detailed in each workout table (see p24 for more on workout tables). The longer you rest between the exercises, the less effective the workout will be and the less likely you are to get the incredible results you want.

THE LAST WORD
Even if you do everything right in the gym and perform the workouts perfectly, you'll still fall short of making positive changes to the way you look if you don't stick to this programme's eating plan. It may be an old fitness cliché, but like all clichés it's based on more than a little truth: you can't out-train a bad diet.

Turn to p20 now to understand how the six-week nutrition plan works and gain all the information you need to succeed.

TIME TO PAY OFF YOUR DEBTS
How high-intensity training helps you burn calories even when you're at rest

Excess post-exercise oxygen consumption, more commonly referred to as EPOC, is the process by which your body increases the amount of oxygen it consumes to repay the oxygen deficit accumulated during a period of intense exercise. This is vital for increased fat loss because it has the effect of increasing your resting metabolic rate (RMR), which is the speed at which your body burns calories while at rest. The higher your RMR, the more calories you burn over the course of a day.

BIG PUSH

The harder you push yourself during training, the greater the oxygen debt you accumulate and the longer it will take your body to return to its pre-training levels.

During this period you burn a greater number of calories than normal and are more likely – if you stick to the nutrition plan – to start using your stores of body fat as fuel.

EATING FOR FAT LOSS

Here's everything you need to know about eating for fat loss

If losing body fat is your main aim, what you do in the kitchen is as important to your chances of success as what you do in the gym. It doesn't matter how hard or effectively you train if you're not as disciplined when sticking to the nutrition plans detailed in this book. Each one is designed to give you the nutrients you need at the right time so you have the energy to train hard and recover well.

The good news is that eating for fat loss isn't complicated, as long as you are disciplined and stick to a number of key rules.

Each meal plan has been built around these considerations, so following them exactly will result in reduced body fat and increased muscle mass. Here are the seven fundamental rules behind the plans.

1 GREEN IS GOOD

Vegetables should be the foundation of your diet and every time you sit down to eat half your plate should be covered in a variety of veg, which contains crucial fibre and lots of other healthy elements. Vegetables do contain carbs, but far less than bread, pasta or potatoes – you'd have to eat half a kilo of asparagus to get the same amount of carbs as in a single wholemeal pitta bread. For more about carbs, see p22.

2 FOCUS ON PROTEIN

Protein is one of the most important components of this nutrition plan. When you eat a high-protein diet, you're generally less hungry, so you eat less and lose weight as a result. It's difficult to eat too much protein but not to get too little, so stick to the serving suggestions in the plans.

EAT VEGETABLES WITH EVERY MEAL AND YOU CAN'T GO WRONG

3 DON'T FEAR FAT

Fat does not make you fat. In fact, you need to consume good-quality fats if you want to burn body fat because this macronutrient has a role in energy expenditure, vitamin storage and making the hormone testosterone, which also increases muscle mass. There's no need to avoid the fats in red meat, avocado and nuts, but you shouldn't eat hydrogenated and trans fats – those found in cakes, biscuits and other processed foods – because these

rule for fat loss? Here's a quick question: which will make you fatter, 2,000 calories from ice cream or 2,000 calories from chicken and veg? Be honest – you know the answer to this already. The intake of the correct macronutrients is ultimately more significant than mere calorie counting. That said, you can't just scoff thousands of calories' worth of healthy food – 5,000 calories from steak is still a lot of calories. The aim is

EGGS ARE AMONG THE BEST SOURCES OF ALL-IMPORTANT PROTEIN

of carcinogens as the wild sort, thanks to cramped conditions and poor-quality feed, while grass-fed beef tends to have much more conjugated linoleic acid and omega 3s than the kind fed on grain and beef tallow. In fact, free range meat and fish is so nutritionally dissimilar to cage-reared that it's basically different food.

> **It may seem strange to eat steak and broccoli first thing, but this will get your metabolism firing to burn body fat**

will derail your fat-loss mission. Plus they're really bad for you.

4 START THE DAY SMART

Think of breakfast like any other meal: you need a blend of protein, fats and veg. It may seem strange to eat steak and broccoli first thing, but such a breakfast will start the supply of quality nutrients to your muscles and get your metabolism firing to burn body fat.

5 CALORIES DON'T COUNT

Still locked into the old-school 'calories in, calories out'

to hit the correct macronutrient numbers to build muscle and burn fat without eating any extra unnecessary calories. So stick to the portion sizes in the meal plans.

6 FREE RANGE IS KEY

Free range animals have a more varied diet and obtain a lot more exercise, which allows the development of more muscle, which in turn means they contain more zinc, vitamins B, A and K, amino acids, iron, selenium, phosphorus and zinc. Farm-raised salmon have also been found to contain up to eight times the level

7 EAT REAL FOOD

If you follow the meal plans in this book you'll follow this by default, but it's a useful rule to remember at all times. Aim to eat only food that grows out of the ground or that once had a face. Alternatively, think like a hunter-gatherer. Ask yourself if a given food would have existed 5,000 years ago. If not, you probably shouldn't eat it. Avoid things containing preservatives that you can't spell or ingredients you wouldn't keep in the kitchen. And eat things that will rot eventually, so that you know they're fresh.

THE TRUTH ABOUT CARBS

Are carbs good or bad when trying to lose weight?
Here's all you need to know

Carbohydrates have a bad rap when it comes to muscle-building and fat loss. But although they spike insulin levels which can result in your body storing more energy as fat, rather than using fat for energy, manipulating your carb intake is one of the most effective ways to get leaner. You just need to be lean enough in the first place to deserve those carbs.

ARE CARBS GOOD OR BAD FOR ME?

It depends on the type, source and, in some cases, the time you consume them, based on your ultimate training aims.

SO WHAT HAPPENS WHEN I EAT CARBS?

Carbs are digested and processed at different rates depending on their structure. In basic terms, the simpler the source – such as sugar – the faster it's digested, with the result being a more rapid rise in blood glucose levels. This in turn prompts your pancreas to release the hormone insulin, which carries glucose – an energy source – into your body's cells where it can be used.

WHAT'S THE DIFFERENCE BETWEEN CARBS?

Carbs are defined by the number of sugar molecules they contain. Complex carbs have three or more sugar molecules. This means they take longer for your body to break down and therefore help to maintain a steady blood glucose level. Simple carbs, on the other hand, elevate blood glucose quickly. Excessive consumption of these can cause short-term problems such as excessive eating and weight gain, as well as serious health issues in the long term.

VEGETABLES CONTAIN COMPLEX CARBS AS WELL AS ESSENTIAL NUTRIENTS AND FIBRE

HOW DO I KNOW WHICH CARBS ARE COMPLEX OR SIMPLE?

The glycaemic index (GI) tells us how quickly each type of carb causes blood glucose levels to rise. Foods are rated one to 100, with 100 causing the fastest rise and the more complex carbs below 60.

❝ Processed sugars provide a lot of calories and can block the body's absorption of other essential nutrients ❞

But this index is only really relevant if the carbs are consumed alone, because eating protein, fats and fibre at the same time will change a carb's GI value. So basing a diet on the GI alone is not advisable.

DO CARBS MAKE YOU FAT?

Not if you eat the right types in the right quantities. Problems arise when too many simple sugars are consumed too regularly. Processed sugars provide a lot of calories but few other nutrients and can block the body's absorption of other essential nutrients.

WHY ARE SIMPLE CARBS SO BAD?

It's easy to eat a lot of simple carbs very quickly and therefore consume too many calories. In addition, eating too many simple carbs results in too much insulin

being released regularly into your system. This affects your insulin resistance and is a precursor of type 2 diabetes, when you have constantly elevated levels of glucose in your blood. Over time, glucose builds up in your organs and nerve endings, which can have serious health implications.

ARE CARBS VITAL TO A FAT-LOSS PROGRAMME?

For elite athletes and those with intense training schedules, carbs have a big role to play, but for the average person wanting to lose weight, consuming the right amount of quality protein, fats, essential nutrients and fluids is far more important. The body can metabolise proteins and fats into glucose in the absence of carbs, if necessary.

WHICH CARBS SHOULD I GO FOR?

Vegetables provide the best bang for your buck. Packed with dense nutrients and fibre, they cause a very stable and manageable rise in blood sugar. If you're training intensively, complex carbs such as rice and potatoes can also help energy levels. Treat wheat with caution – many people have problems digesting it efficiently.

TAKEAWAY TIPS

Here are the key points to remember when eating for fat loss

ORGANISATION IS EVERYTHING
To stick to the meal plans in this book you need to be organised. Buy in bulk to reduce costs and batch-cook and freeze meals so they are ready when you need them. If you're not organised you may be tempted to grab a convenient sandwich or snack, or even to order a takeaway.

AVOID TEMPTATIONS
Before you start this programme empty your cupboards of all the foods you're not going to need for the next six weeks. If these products are sitting there tempting you to eat them, you are more likely to.

If they're not, you can't. And bin all your takeaway menus.

BANISH THE BOOZE
Drinking alcohol is one of the most harmful things you can do when trying to lose weight or build muscle. It's high in calories and provides no essential nutrients, plus your body prioritises the task of metabolising alcohol ahead of burning fat or building muscle. Plus a few drinks at night means you are less likely to stick to your diet and focus fully at your next training session. Avoid alcohol to get the best results possible.

SESSION STRATEGY

Discover how each week's workouts will result in a leaner you

Following this fat-loss plan could not be easier. Each of the six weeks has been given its own chapter, which contains details of what you need to eat that week and when, as well as the week's four training sessions – three weight-training workouts and one high-intensity cardio session.

All you need to do is stick to the seven-day menu and perform each of the workouts in order, leaving at least a day's rest between each of the three weight-training sessions.

A good way to do this is to do the first workout on a Monday, the second on a Wednesday and the third on a Friday. You can then complete the week with the intensive cardio session over the weekend, before starting the next cycle on the following Monday.

WORKOUT FOCUS

The first workout each week works all the major muscles of your upper body, the second concentrates on your lower body and the third is a total-body session.

Each workout comprises eight different exercises split into two sets of four moves, which are known as 'giant sets'. A giant set is four or more exercises performed back to back with little or no rest taken between each exercise. You only get an extended rest after completing the final rep of the fourth move.

After that rest period, you start again and repeat the process until the required number of sets have been completed. You then

> **Each workout comprises eight different exercises split into two sets of four moves, which are known as giant sets**

move on to the second giant set and repeat the process. The exact rest periods you should take are detailed in the workout tables for each week, along with the number of sets, reps and tempo for each move (see box, right, for details).

At the end of each of these three workouts you'll find a suggested Fat-Loss Finisher. This is a high-intensity move that has been included to really push your body out of its comfort zone, send

your heart rate soaring and burn as much fat as possible. The form guides for these exercises can be found on pp172-177.

LIFT SMART

Weight lifting has a number of key benefits if fat loss is your primary objective of working out. The main one is that it works your muscles very hard, which has the effect of releasing a number of important hormones, specifically the male sex hormone testosterone and human growth hormone. Both of these instruct your body to burn excess fat stores and build lean muscle tissue.

Another key benefit is that taking little or no rest between lifts quickly sends your heart rate soaring, forcing your heart and lungs to work at near-maximum capacity to get enough blood and oxygen to your muscles. However, if you work out intensively enough your body can't

EXERCISE ORDER
This is the order in which you perform
the four moves of each giant set.

SETS
The number of sets you
perform of each move.

REPS
The number of times you perform an exercise
in each set before moving on to the next move.

WEEK ONE ▶ UPPER BODY

	EXERCISE	SETS	REPS	TEMPO	REST
1A	Dumbbell bench press	3	12	2010	10sec
1B	Dumbbell shoulder press	3	12	2010	10sec
1C	Dumbbell flye	3	10	2010	10sec
1D	Dumbbell biceps curl	3	10	2010	90sec
2A	Dumbbell bent-over row	3	12	2110	10sec
2B	Dumbbell bent-over flye	3	12	2010	10sec
2C	Underhand lat pull-down	3	10	2110	10sec
2D	Seated row	3	10	2010	90sec

WORKOUT 1

•• Perform the first sets of 1A, 1B, 1C and 1D, taking 10 seconds' rest
between each. Then rest for 90 seconds and repeat until all three
sets are completed.

•• Perform the first sets of 2A, 2B, 2C and 2D, taking 10 seconds' rest
between each. Then rest for 90 seconds and repeat until all three
sets are completed.

TEMPO
The speed of the lift. If you want to see the best results, it's vital you stick to the right tempo.
The first number is the speed in seconds of the lowering portion of a lift, such as lowering
the bar to your chest in a bench press. The second is the pause at the bottom, the third is
the speed of lifting the weight and the fourth is the pause between reps. An X means you
should do that part of the move as quickly as possible while maintaining perfect form.

REST
The amount of time
you should take between
each part of the giant
set before moving
on to the next.

get enough oxygen, resulting in an 'oxygen debt'. This is critical to you achieving your goals, because the greater an oxygen deficit you can create, the more fat you'll burn.

This oxygen repayment process is known as excess post-exercise oxygen consumption, or EPOC, and getting oxygen levels back to normal causes your body's metabolism – the rate at which it burns calories – to rise, which

is why fat stores are broken down and burned as energy. The increased rate of calorie burning continues for up to 48 hours after your session has ended, so you burn fat for longer.

The final advantage is that working out intensively forces your heart and lungs to work as hard as your muscles, so you gain health benefits that will lead make these key organs more efficient, resulting

in even greater fitness levels.

The beauty of the final high-intensity cardio workout each week is that short, sharp bursts of all-out effort replicate all the key benefits of the three weight training sessions. The result? You get leaner, stronger and fitter every time you train.

TURN OVER
for our easy-to-follow
table explaining the order in
which you should perform
the workouts in this
fat-loss training plan

PROGRESS REPORT

Your easy-to-follow quick-reference chart of all the workouts and cardio sessions you must perform over the next six weeks

WORKOUT	MUSCLE GROUP	WORKOUT TABLE	FORM GUIDES
WEEK 1			
1	UPPER BODY	p56	p58
2	LOWER BODY	p57	p62
3	TOTAL BODY	p57	p66
4	HIGH-INTENSITY CARDIO	n/a	p70
WEEK 2			
1	UPPER BODY	p76	p78
2	LOWER BODY	p77	p82
3	TOTAL BODY	p77	p86
4	HIGH-INTENSITY CARDIO	n/a	p90
WEEK 3			
1	UPPER BODY	p96	p98
2	LOWER BODY	p97	p102
3	TOTAL BODY	p97	p106
4	HIGH-INTENSITY CARDIO	n/a	p110
WEEK 4			
1	UPPER BODY	p116	p118
2	LOWER BODY	p117	p122
3	TOTAL BODY	p117	p126
4	HIGH-INTENSITY CARDIO	n/a	p130
WEEK 5			
1	UPPER BODY	p136	p138
2	LOWER BODY	p137	p142
3	TOTAL BODY	p137	p146
4	HIGH-INTENSITY CARDIO	n/a	p150
WEEK 6			
1	UPPER BODY	p156	p158
2	LOWER BODY	p157	p162
3	TOTAL BODY	p157	p166
4	HIGH-INTENSITY CARDIO	n/a	p170

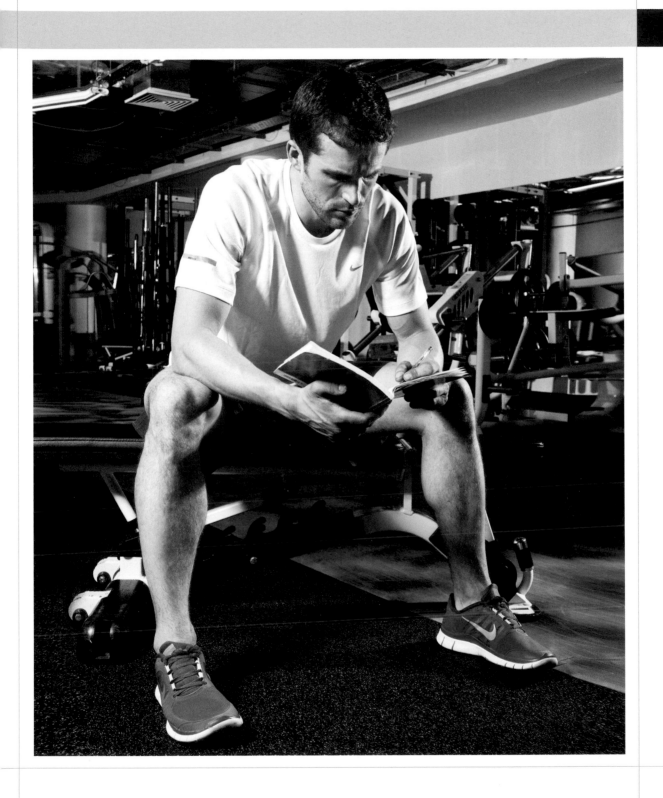

GYM BASICS

Simple answers to the most common training questions

Q **I've tried and failed to lose weight in the past. Why will it work now?**
If your previous efforts have been unsuccessful it has nothing to do with your body being resistant to exercise and everything to do with your approach. In other words, you probably didn't have a realistic goal, a focused and progressive training plan or eat the right foods at the right time – or a combination of all three. Anyone can lose body fat to transform significantly the way they look but that won't happen overnight. But the six-week training and nutrition plan in this book, if followed without fault, will give you a better body.

Q **Can I turn fat into muscle?**
No, fat and muscle are two totally different types of tissue and it's impossible to turn one into the other. Muscle is active tissue that burns calories, while fat tissue stores excess energy. The right training programme will burn off these fat stores and build new muscle tissue, giving the

appearance that one has turned into the other, but that isn't the case.

Q **How many times a week do I need train?**
This programme requires you to work out four times a week. This plan consists of three weight-training sessions and one high-intensity cardio session each week. You need to leave at least one day's rest between the weights sessions to give your body time to recover.

Q **How closely do I need to follow the workout plan?**
To the letter. Every workout has been designed to elicit a fat-burning response and forms an important part of a structured and progressive training plan that will significantly reduce the amount of fat you carry. Do the workouts in order for the best results possible.

Q **What about sticking to the sets, reps, tempo and rest numbers detailed?**
These are crucial too. You need to complete all the sets and reps at

the correct tempo while sticking to the rest periods between the moves. Failure to do so will limit the success of your fat-loss journey.

Q **What if I can't complete all the sets and reps?**
If this is the case, the weight you're lifting is too heavy and you need to reduce it. This programme isn't about lifting the heaviest weight possible, but exposing your muscles and cardiovascular system to the right amount of stress to make your body take positive steps towards becoming fitter and leaner.

Q **How do I know which weights to use?**
At first there will be a little bit of trial and error because the amount of weight you should be lifting will depend on a number of factors unique to you, such as age and training experience. It's always best to choose a light weight if you are unsure and stick to the reps at the right tempo. If you can complete the set with ease, you should increase the weight next time.

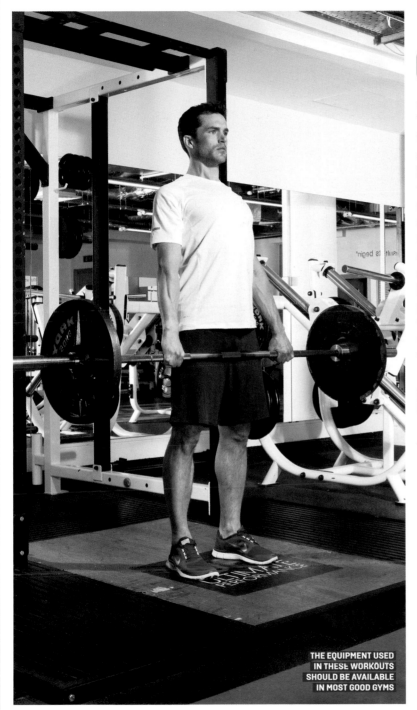

THE EQUIPMENT USED IN THESE WORKOUTS SHOULD BE AVAILABLE IN MOST GOOD GYMS

Q What should I do if my gym doesn't have the equipment used in some of the exercises in this plan?

This programme has been designed to be as easy and efficient to follow as possible, with many moves in each of the giant sets using the same piece of equipment so you don't waste time moving around the gym between moves. However, depending on the quality of your gym, some may not have exactly every single bit of kit you need. That's not a problem: just swap those moves for ones that target the same muscles which you can do with the equipment available to you.

Q Why do I need to do a Fat-Loss Finisher after each weight-training session?

All three weight-training sessions each week are designed to build lean muscle mass and reduce body fat to radically transform your physique so you look stronger and leaner. The Fat-Loss Finisher at the end of each of these three sessions is designed to push your body even further out of its comfort zone to elicit the best fat-burning response possible by increasing the oxygen debt your body needs to repay (see p16 for details) and result in the right hormonal response to encourage the building of new muscle and the burning of fat cells.

FOOD RULES

The principles behind your six-week fat-loss nutrition plan

What you eat and when is critical to your success of building a leaner body. Which is why we have made following the six-week nutrition plan in this book as easy as possible.

At the start of each weekly chapter there is a seven-day meal plan for you to follow. To ensure you stick to the schedule, look at week one before you start and fill your cupboards, fridge and freezer with all the foods you'll need that week. Not having the right foods to hand will make it impossible to stick to the plan and have you reaching for the takeaway menus.

These are the rules on which this nutrition plan is based.

1 LEAN MEAT FOR BREAKFAST

Eating lean meat for breakfast is one the best things you can do when wanting to lose weight. Meat allows for a slow and steady rise in blood sugar levels, which keeps you feeling fuller for longer so you aren't tempted to reach for sweets to boost energy by mid-morning. It also provides a big dose of protein first thing, which helps repair the damage done to your muscles through training, and improves focus so you are more determined to stick to the diet plan throughout the rest of the day.

2 PROTEIN WITH EVERY MEAL

As we mentioned on p20, people on a high-protein diet find it easier to lose weight, and it's almost impossible to eat too much. Almost every meal in each plan contains a source of high-quality lean protein to ensure you get enough each day to repair your muscles, while burning fat.

3 PLENTY OF FRESH VEGETABLES

Along with protein, vegetables should form a significant part of each meal — roughly half, in fact. Veg is high in antioxidants and many essential vitamins and minerals to keep you fighting fit, and full of fibre, which will also help you feel full long after eating. Vegetables are also very low in calories.

4 CARBS AROUND TRAINING

Most of the carbs in the meal plans are to be eaten around your workouts. This is because carbs allow you to recover from training faster, and it's important you are fully energised for each session so you can push yourself. All these carbs rank low on the glycaemic index, which means they don't raise blood sugar levels too rapidly so your body is constantly in the best state to burn fat.

5 PLENTY OF WATER

Dehydration leads to poor focus and lack of motivation. These things can cause you to make poor food choices and perform badly in the gym, so aim to drink two to three litres a day, and more on training days. Water also flushes toxins and waste from your body, making you more efficient and helping you get fitter and leaner.

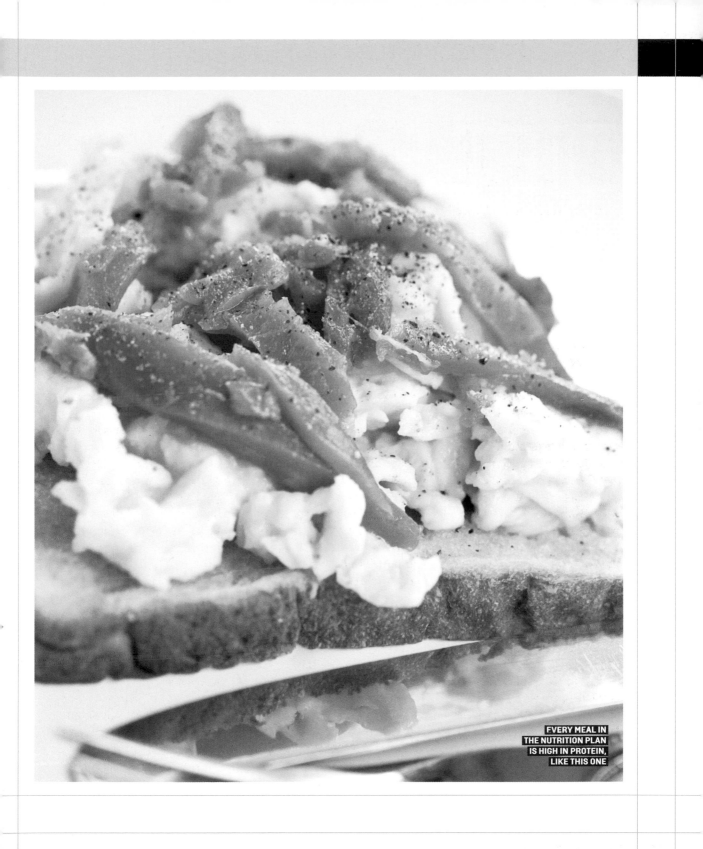

EVERY MEAL IN
THE NUTRITION PLAN
IS HIGH IN PROTEIN,
LIKE THIS ONE

DIET BASICS

Discover the answers to common questions about this meal plan

Q How closely do I need to follow this programme's weekly meal plans?
You need to follow them as closely as possible. Each meal plan has been designed to provide you with just the right amount of nutrients to allow your body to recover from training so you can attack the next session at 100%, without giving you any more than is necessary. Falling to stick to the key principles behind each day's diet will undo much of the hard work you put in at the gym.

Q Some of the meals aren't exactly exciting my tastebuds. Is there anything I do about that?
The majority of your meals over the next six weeks will be based around lean sources of protein and fresh vegetables. What's not to like? If this is a radical departure from your normal diet, this is a good thing because you are likely to see results faster.

You need to remember that for the next six weeks you are eating for a better body, not your tastebuds, so try to enjoy the new diet plan because it will make you thinner. If you do find the meals too bland to stomach, you can add spices, chilli flakes, garlic and herbs to give them some flavour and kick.

Q I find that I'm often hungry before I go to bed. Is this OK?
It may be that you experience a few more hunger pangs than you're used to when eating to lose weight, but this isn't necessarily a bad thing. It may simply be because your body is used to being fed more often and with foods that you now need to avoid.

This programme's weekly meal plans have been designed to provide the right amount of protein and fat each day so you have enough energy to train hard and recover fully without leaving you hungry, because any more food than is absolutely necessary could be stored as fat. If you find you're hungry a lot of the time, you can increase the amount of meat and veg you eat, especially in the evenings.

Q Is there anything I can do to make sure I stick to the meal plans?
Organisation is key. You need to know what you're eating and when for the following seven days so you have all the supplies in your home and ready to eat. If you don't have what you need at hand, you're far more likely to stray from the plan and eat convenience foods that are high in carbs, especially sugar. Whenever possible, spend some time each evening preparing the next day's meals and snacks – that's one of the best ways to stay on the right path.

Q How can I reduce the cost of my weekly shopping?
Vegetables are inexpensive, but lean meat can be pricey. However, buying in bulk can significantly reduce your expenditure on food and is easy to do on this plan because all your meals for the next six weeks are mapped out for you. Another advantage of shopping this way is you can batch cook and freeze meals for later in the programme.

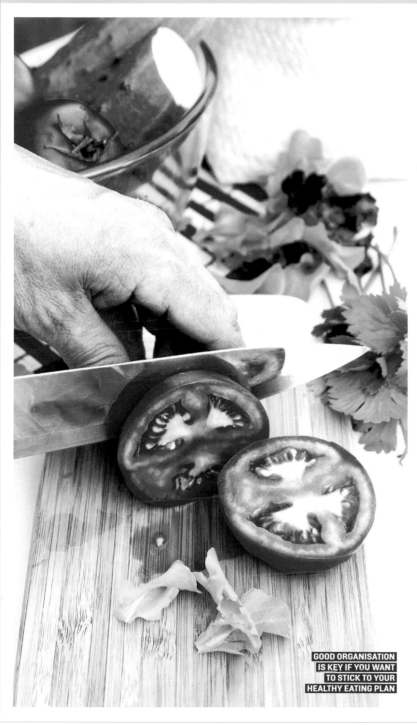

GOOD ORGANISATION IS KEY IF YOU WANT TO STICK TO YOUR HEALTHY EATING PLAN

Q Can I drink alcohol over the next six weeks?

If you want to achieve the best results possible, you should steer clear of alcohol. There are many reasons for this. Alcohol is just empty calories – it contains energy but very few nutrients. Your body prioritises processing alcohol over other things, such as burning fat and building muscle. You're less likely to stick to your diet plan when under the influence of alcohol because it affects blood sugar levels and stimulates your appetite. It can be so tempting to skip the next day's training session if you're hungover.

If you can't avoid alcohol entirely, stick to the very occasional glass of red wine, but remember that every drink you have will limit the extent of your transformation.

Q How important are supplements to my progress?

Not as important as sticking to the meal plans. Supplements are just that – they supplement a varied and well-balanced diet to help you on your way to a better body. Some supplements, such as whey protein and omega 3 fatty acids, are more important than others when fat loss is your primary objective. For our full round-up of which supplements you may need and when best to take them, turn to p34.

SUPER SUPPS

Take the right supplements at the right time for greater gains

Whether you regularly pack a protein shake in your gym bag or just chug the occasional isotonic sports drink, chances are you've used supplements at one time or another. The trouble is, the whole process can get a bit confusing – with every supplier claiming its brand is better filtered, or more efficient, or will pack on more muscle – to the point where you feel as if you need a degree in chemistry to understand what you're putting into your body.

Don't worry, help is at hand. The science behind some supplements may be slightly baffling, but over the next few pages we've put together the definitive guide to the latest developments in supplement science: what you need, when you need it, why you need it and what – if any – are its potential pitfalls.

It's possible you'll find something to send your training gains through the roof, or you might just learn a bit more about the stuff you're already using. Either way, next time you put in a hard day at the gym, you'll know you're getting the nutritional back-up you need.

WHAT SUPP?
We answer the most frequently asked supplement questions

Q Is it not possible to get all the nutrition I need from my daily diet?
Yes, if you really watch what you eat. Having said that, you may find that sometimes getting the optimum amount of certain substances for your training means eating a lot. For example, consuming the amount of creatine many trainers recommend would mean eating an awful lot of beef, which would not be feasible in most cases. Use supplements to fill the gaps in your diet, but don't rely on them to counteract bad eating habits.

Q Should I take supplements on the days I'm not training?
Yes. You get stronger as you recover from exercise, so making sure you're getting enough nutrients on your rest days is essential.

Q Should I be waking in the middle of the night to take supplements?
Almost definitely not. You might have heard about bodybuilders getting up at 3am to neck a quick shake, but as soon as you're awake for more than three seconds you disrupt the production of melatonin, which is one of the most important hormones in getting to sleep. You're better off having some nice slow-digesting protein – such as raw nuts, cottage cheese or a casein shake – before bed.

Q Are supplements safe?
Since sports supplements are technically classified as food, they aren't subject to the same strict manufacturing, safety testing or labelling as licensed medicines, so there's no guarantee they're living up to their claims. The EU is currently looking into the situation with a view to introducing stricter guidelines, but in the meantime it's up to individual manufacturers to maintain the quality of their own products. Look for supplements that are ISO17025 certified, which means

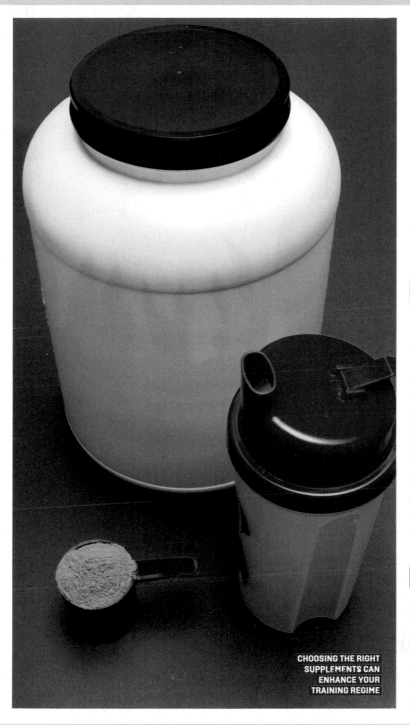

CHOOSING THE RIGHT SUPPLEMENTS CAN ENHANCE YOUR TRAINING REGIME

TOP TIP
A post-workout protein shake will rebuild your muscles faster

they've been subjected to rigorous checks during their production.

Q Could taking supplements result in me failing a drugs test?

Maybe. If you're a serious enough sportsman to be tested, you must be careful. A survey conducted by an International Olympic Committee-accredited laboratory in Cologne looked for steroids in 634 supplements and found 15 per cent contained substances that would cause a failed drug test, although none contained actual steroids. If you're concerned, consult a registered nutritionist or dietician, or talk to your sports federation.

Q Can I get ripped without working out if I take the right supplements?

Sadly, no. Anyone who tells you otherwise is fibbing. Eat right, train hard, tailor your supplement use to your goals and choose well-researched and tested products, and you'll see the results you want.

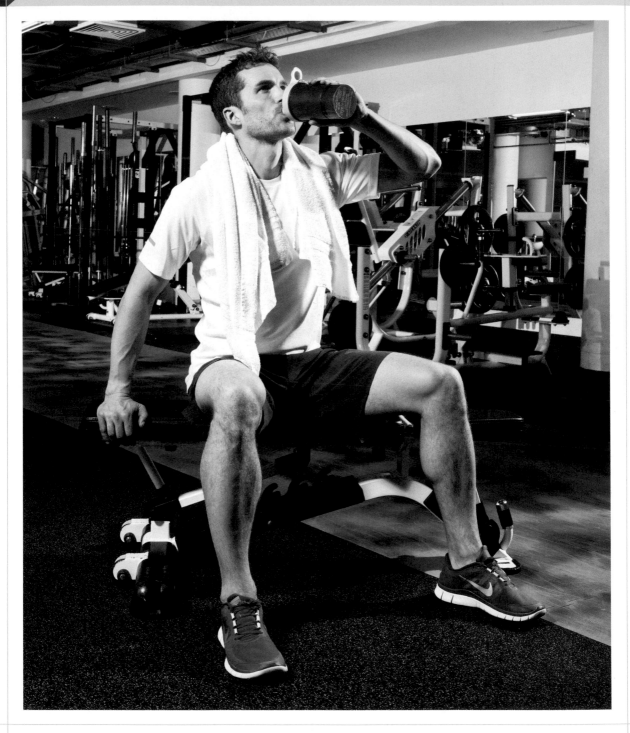

MUSCLE UP

Discover the best supplements for adding lean muscle mass

WHEY PROTEIN

WHAT The post-workout protein

WHY Whey is a fast-release protein, which means it's digested quickly and gets into your bloodstream – and your muscles – fast. What you consume after training is one of the most important meals you eat, so make sure you buy a high-quality whey protein.

HOW Your muscles are most receptive to nutrients as soon as you finish training, so drink a protein shake as soon as you've completed your final rep. Aim for a minimum of 30g of whey protein powder.

CASEIN

WHAT The bedtime protein

WHY Chances are you're already getting a fair hit of casein as it makes up around 80% of cow's milk. It's a slow-release protein, which means you get a 'drip-feed' effect over a longer period. This makes it unsuitable for taking straight after a workout when you need an instant hit of nutrients, but it's ideal for consuming just before you go to bed.

HOW Have it in a shake with either water or milk before turning in for the night. This will mean your muscles receive quality protein while you are sleeping, which is when your muscles are repaired and rebuilt.

BCAA

WHAT The muscle pill

WHY Branched-chain amino acids, or BCAA, are the best supplement to take during workouts because they help to keep a steady supply of proteins flowing into your muscles. This helps with muscle building as it reduces the amount of muscle loss during exercise and improves protein synthesis, the process by which new muscle tissue is built. BCAAs can also help to prevent muscle loss during periods of intermittent fasting.

HOW Take up to 2g between every set during a long workout.

CREATINE

WHAT The back-up generator

WHY Your body metabolises creatine into ATP, which is used for every initial muscle movement. It's therefore vital to have adequate supplies when you're doing heavy, high-intensity workouts in order to deliver the required energy to your muscles. In other words, creatine helps you lift harder for longer.

HOW Take 2-10g in your post-workout shake to replenish lost stores. Alternatively, split your dose and have half before your workout and half afterwards. And make sure you drink plenty of water with it: creatine is hygroscopic, which means it will suck water into your muscles and can leave you dehydrated.

LEUCINE

WHAT The muscle booster

WHY The most anabolic amino acid, leucine can independently stimulate insulin secretion and muscle protein synthesis, enhancing the muscle-building process. At 11%, whey protein is very high in leucine content, which is one reason it's so effective as a post-workout elixir.

HOW Taking a 5g dose of leucine after training and between meals can increase the anabolic – or muscle-building – effect of the foods you eat, especially when you're consuming protein sources that are low in leucine and which therefore might not stimulate maximum muscle protein synthesis on their own.

THE BEST OF THE REST

Use these supplements for better health and performance

FISH OIL

WHAT The wonder fluid

WHY It's important to include omega 3 fats in your diet for health reasons, and a supplement can help you to maintain a good ratio of omega 3 to omega 6 – most of us consume too much of the latter. Studies have shown fish oil supplementation results in decreased body fat and reduced inflammation. It has also been linked with increased serotonin levels, more focus in training and less stress.

HOW Take a spoonful with meals. Most authorities recommend 1-4g a day, depending on how much oily fish is already included in your diet.

GLUTAMINE

WHAT The gut calmer

WHY This amino acid should be present in your body, but if you have problems with your digestion or are training hard, a supplement can help to strengthen the lining of your gut and help protein synthesis.

HOW There are several ways to take this, depending on your goals. Take 10g in water on an empty stomach to aid gut function or 10g after your workout to help replenish glutamine stores. If you're on a low-carb diet, take 30g after your workout to enhance glycogen replenishment.

GREEN TEA

WHAT The diet drink

WHY This is one of the best natural fat-burners around and can give your metabolism a jolt. Green tea is also packed with antioxidants and has been linked to the prevention of a range of conditions, from heart disease to Alzheimer's.

HOW Drink instead of your regular tea or diet soft drink.

HCL

WHAT The digestion helper

WHY Hydrochloric acid (HCL) is the acid responsible for digesting and breaking down animal protein in your stomach. Taking a supplement will ensure you're actually getting the benefit of all the protein you're eating. If you aren't digesting and breaking down nutrients properly in your gut, then all other supplements and healthy foods could simply be wasted as you won't be able to absorb them effectively.

HOW Take one or two tablets with each meal.

L-CARNITINE

WHAT The fat shredder

WHY If burning fat during a workout is your priority, first you need to mobilise it. L-carnitine is an amino acid responsible for transporting fatty acids into the mitochondria, our cells' energy powerhouses.

HOW Take a single dose of 500-3,000mg before your workout to make sure you transport the maximum amount of available fat for fuel during exercise. It's especially

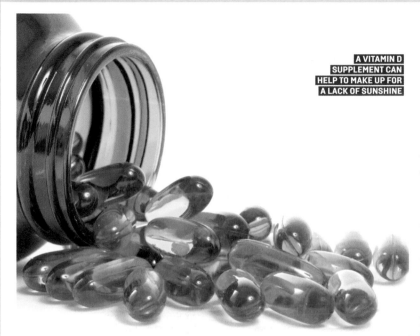

WHAT The sun substitute
WHY You should get your vitamin D from the sun, but that's a forlorn hope for the average deskbound Briton – 20 minutes' exposure is enough in the summer, but according to the National Institute of Health it's impossible to get enough come the winter. Deficiency is common and linked to lower strength levels and increased body fat. It has also been associated with a number of diseases, including cancer, diabetes and depression.
HOW Supplements are available in tablet form or as an oral spray. Official government recommendations are low – aim for 3,000IU a day, which has been proved safe in multiple studies. It's fat-soluble, so take it with a meal.

– taking magnesium on an empty stomach can lead to diarrhoea and an upset stomach. Or you can use a magnesium spray or lotion.

MULTIVITAMINS

WHAT The back-up plan
WHY Although you shouldn't rely on them to make up for a bad diet, a quality multivitamin can help to fill in the gaps in an otherwise solid eating plan. Deficiencies in vitamins can cause mood swings, depression, lethargy and exhaustion, but taking a daily dose will keep you on the up and focused on your goals. There is also evidence a multivitamin can help you recover from a tough workout.
HOW Try to take multivitamins at a consistent time of the day. It makes sense to take them before a meal, with a glass of water to aid absorption of their micronutrients.

ZINC

WHAT The masculine mineral
WHY Zinc is vital for your health and immune system. Our bodies aren't able to store it so you need to top up regularly.
HOW The RDA for zinc is 11mg for adult males – take no more than 40mg per day. Don't take it with coffee or foods containing phytates – such as wholegrains – because they can block its absorption. For the best benefits, take it with animal proteins as they promote absorption.

useful to take if you're training while fasting or on a low-carb diet, when fat oxidation is maximised.

MAGNESIUM

WHAT The body calmer
WHY Every organ needs magnesium, especially the heart, muscles and kidneys. If you skimp on this vital mineral you can experience anxiety, sleep problems and irritability. Magnesium also helps to maintain a normal heart rhythm and aids in the body's energy production.
HOW Stick to the recommended dose of less than 350mg a day and remember to take it with food

KNOW YOUR MUSCLES

There are over 600 muscles in the human body. These are the major ones you'll be targeting during your workouts

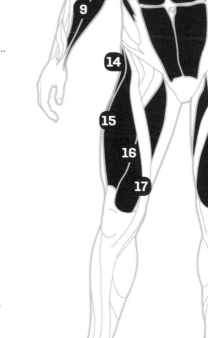

DELTOIDS
1 Medial deltoid (middle)

2 Anterior deltoid (front)

PECTORALS
3 Pectoralis major

4 Pectoralis minor (beneath the pectoralis major)

5 Serratus anterior

BICEPS
6 Biceps brachii

7 Brachialis

FOREARMS
8 Brachioradialis

9 Flexor carpi radialis

ABDOMINALS
10 Rectus abdominis

11 External obliques

12 Internal obliques (beneath the external obliques)

13 Transverse abdominis (beneath the internal obliques)

QUADRICEPS
14 Vastus lateralis

15 Rectus femoris

16 Vastus intermedius (beneath the rectus femoris)

17 Vastus medialis

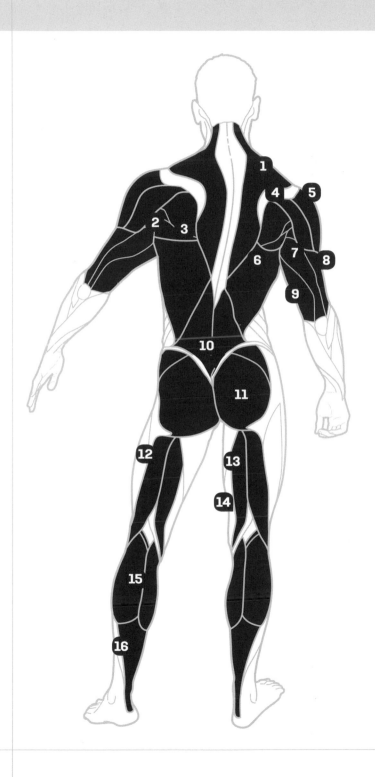

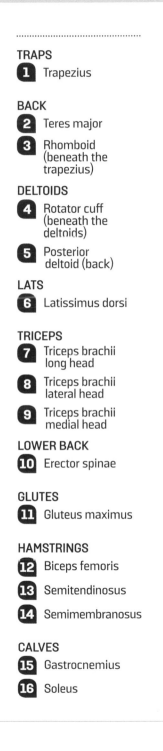

TRAPS

1 Trapezius

BACK

2 Teres major

3 Rhomboid (beneath the trapezius)

DELTOIDS

4 Rotator cuff (beneath the deltoids)

5 Posterior deltoid (back)

LATS

6 Latissimus dorsi

TRICEPS

7 Triceps brachii long head

8 Triceps brachii lateral head

9 Triceps brachii medial head

LOWER BACK

10 Erector spinae

GLUTES

11 Gluteus maximus

HAMSTRINGS

12 Biceps femoris

13 Semitendinosus

14 Semimembranosus

CALVES

15 Gastrocnemius

16 Soleus

BIGGER & STRONGER

The simple science behind adding muscle mass

48 HOURS
The minimum amount of time you should leave between training sessions focusing on the same muscle group

Your body is a clever old thing. The process of muscle growth is essentially your body's response to the stress of weight training. It thinks, 'That was hard. I'd better do something about it so it's not as difficult next time.'

When you perform resistance exercises, microscopic tears occur in your muscles. Your body responds to this 'microtrauma' by overcompensating: the damaged tissue is repaired and more is added, making your muscles bigger and stronger so the risk of future damage is minimised. This also means over time you need to increase steadily the weight you lift, because your muscles quickly adapt to deal with the stress.

It's thought this damage to your muscle fibres is the reason for delayed onset muscle soreness, or DOMS, the symptoms of which include muscle soreness and stiffness in the days after a tough workout. That's why you should leave at least 48 hours between sessions that target the same muscle group. If you train those muscles again before they've had time to repair and rebuild you risk overtraining, which can result in reduced gains and injury.

ANATOMY OF A MUSCLE
Discover what your muscles are made of

Muscles are made up of bundles of fibres contained in protective sheaths called fascia, which are then themselves bundled together.

The biggest bundle is the muscle itself. Next are the fascicles, which contain muscle fibres. These are then divided into myofibrils, which are divided into myofilaments, made up from chains of sarcomeres.

1 TENDON
Strong, connective tissue connecting muscle to bone.

2 EPIMYSIUM
A layer of connective tissue encasing the entire muscle.

3 ENDOMYSIUM
Connective tissue covering the muscle fibres. Also contains capillaries (tiny blood vessels) and nerves.

4 PERIMYSIUM
A layer of connective tissue that bundles between ten and several hundred individual muscle fibres to create fascicles.

5 FASCICLE
A bundle of individual muscle fibres.

6 MYOFILAMENTS
These are the smallest fibre bundles, made up of sarcomeres, the basic unit of a muscle.

7 MUSCLE FIBRE
Individual muscle fibres come in two main types: type 1 or slow-twitch, suited to endurance because they are slow to fatigue; and type 2 or fast-twitch, which are quick to fatigue and therefore suited to fast, explosive movements.

There are several key stages in the process that breaks down muscle fibres before they can be rebuilt stronger

WARM-UP
As your heart rate increases, blood is pumped into your muscles, warming them up and allowing them to extend fully. The blood also supplies the muscle fibres with oxygen.

UNDER TENSION
At the start of a rep, your muscles are under tension and stretched. As a result more blood is pumped into the protective sheaths of the muscle fibres, supplying even more oxygen and nutrients.

INITIAL SPARK
As you lift a weight, your central nervous system relays this to the nerves in the sheaths around the muscle fibres, telling the fibres to contract. If you do the exercise correctly your muscles will activate in a particular sequence, which your nervous system adapts to. As you repeat the workout, your nerves get more efficient, allowing you to do more. This is the first adaptation caused by weightlifting.

CHEMICAL REACTION
Adenosine triphosphate (ATP) is the immediate energy source for these muscle contractions. It is broken down within the body's cells to release energy. The cells' creatine, phosphate and glycogen reserves are also converted into ATP. This process creates lactic acid as a by-product.

FEEL THE BURN
Once the glycogen stores in your cells have been depleted and lactic acid starts to builds up the muscle can't work efficiently, so you have to rest. As you do so, aerobic (oxygen-based) muscle respiration occurs, processing the lactic acid back into glycogen and giving you an energy source for the next set.

SUCCESSFUL FAILURE
As you reach failure on the last set of a given exercise, your fast-twitch muscle fibres are completely fatigued. Microscopic tears ('microtears') occur in the myofilaments, the smallest fibre bundles in your muscles.

REPAIR AND GROWTH
Your muscles start to grow during the post-workout repair process. Your body fixes the microtears by adding the amino acids actin and myosin to the myofilaments, which also causes them to grow. Your muscles adapt to store more glycogen too, so there's more energy for the next workout. This also has the happy side effect of making the muscles slightly bigger.

❽ BLOOD VESSEL
Part of the body's circulatory system, blood vessels come in three types: arteries, responsible for transporting oxygenated blood away from the heart to the organs and tissues; capillaries, which enable the exchange of nutrients and waste products between the blood and tissues; and veins, which transport deoxygenated blood from the capillaries back to the heart.

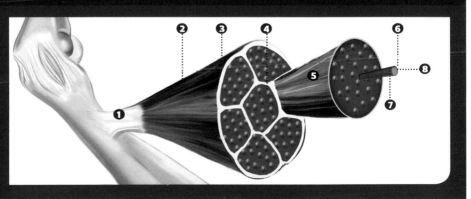

HOW FAT IS BURNED

The simple science behind how your body burns fat for fuel

For many years, most people have believed the key to losing fat is to burn more calories than they consume. But while calorie consumption should be monitored, losing weight isn't quite as simple as that.

Different macronutrients – protein, carbohydrates and fat – have different effects on your body. A high-carb diet means your body always has enough energy to burn without needing to tap into fat stores. On the other hand, restricting your carb intake forces your body to use fat for fuel. So while ensuring you don't eat too many calories is important, lowering your daily amount of carbs is critical to getting your body into the right environment to burn fat.

FAT BURNING MADE SIMPLE

Here's how this training and diet plan will burn body fat to get you into shape.

1 When your blood sugar levels are low, because you're not eating many carbs or have gone a while without eating, the pancreas responds by releasing the hormone glucagon to raise them.

2 To do this, glucagon causes free fatty acids from fat cells to be released into the bloodstream.

3 These fatty acids are transported to your liver, where they're converted into glucose that your muscles and brain can use as fuel.

BODY-FAT RANGES

The American Council on Exercise classification of body-fat percentages for men and women

DESCRIPTION	WOMEN	MEN
Essential fat only	10–13%	2–5%
Athlete	14–20%	6–13%
Fit	21–24%	14–17%
Average	25–31%	18–24%
Obese	32%+	25%+

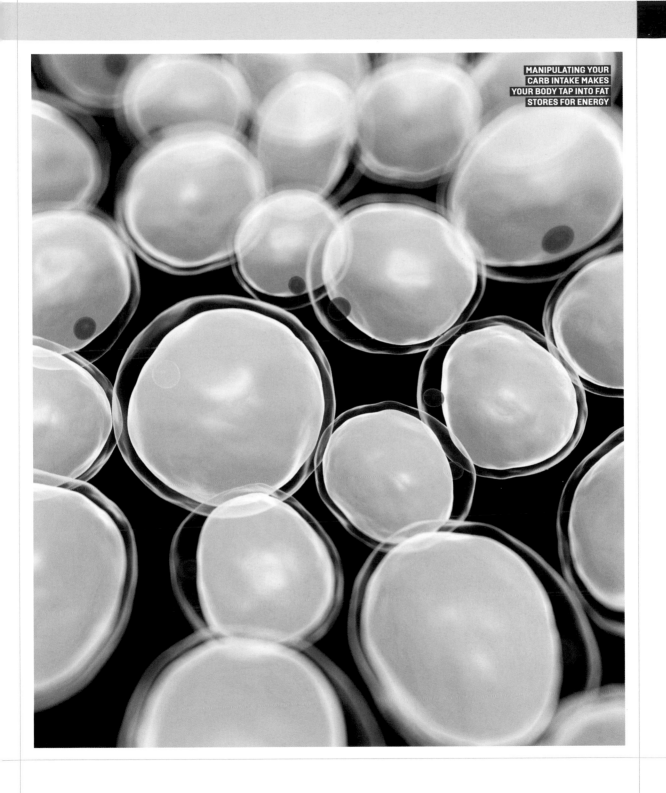

MANIPULATING YOUR
CARB INTAKE MAKES
YOUR BODY TAP INTO FAT
STORES FOR ENERGY

BEFORE YOU GET STARTED

Straightforward answers to your last-minute queries

Q Can anyone follow this plan?

Absolutely. Because you choose which weights you lift, the training plan is suitable for all fitness abilities, whether you're new to exercise, getting back into it after a break or an experienced trainer. All you need to do is follow the training plan and ensure you perform each exercise according to the pictorial demonstrations and detailed written form guides. Find a weight that is suitable for your level of experience and stick to the sets, reps, tempo and rest periods detailed.

Q I have a lot of time commitments. Is this a problem?

Each weekly training plan contains just four sessions, each one lasting less than an hour, so you don't need to find much time each week to make giant strides towards a better body. It may be the case that you need to get up an hour earlier to exercise before work, but this is a small sacrifice for just six weeks considering that your reward will be a stronger, leaner physique.

Q Should I do other exercise on top of this plan?

The key to losing weight is to eat smart and train intensively for a short period of time. This plan has been designed to be all you need to lose fat and training on top it may result in your become tired, fatigued and irritable, so try to avoid any intensive exercise outside of the regime in this book. However, getting out and about more regularly throughout the day – even it's just for a quick walk – will all add up to making you fitter and healthier.

Q I feel lethargic all the time. Is there something wrong?

At first you may struggle for energy because it's likely you haven't trained this way before. It can also take a little time for your body to adjust to a high-protein, low-carb diet, especially if your diet was previously built around eating a lot of carbs. Don't worry – stick to the programme and it will soon become easier as your body adapts to the changes.

Q My muscles really ache in the days after a workout. Is this normal?

Having sore muscles in the day or two after a hard session is normal and proves you've pushed your muscles out of their comfort zone. This is critical to achieving the best results. Don't worry, the stiffness won't last. It's just your muscles going through the repair process that results in them being more efficient at exercise.

IMPORTANT Always consult your GP before starting a new exercise programme

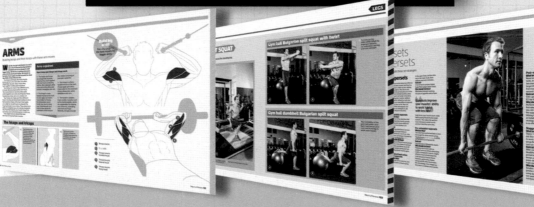

GLOSSARY

Explanations of some common workout terms

COMPOUND LIFT

An exercise involving movement in two or more joints, such as the squat (hip and knee) and shoulder press (shoulder and elbow). Such lifts should form the basis of all programmes where increasing muscle size and strength are the aims because they recruit more of the muscle fibres responsible for those attributes.

FAILURE

When you're unable to lift the weight with correct form on the final rep of your set. This shocks your muscles into growing back bigger and stronger.

GIANT SETS

Four or more moves done back to back with little or no rest between them. They allow you to train with more volume in a shorter period. Each weights session in this plan is made up of two giant sets.

HYPERTROPHY

Greek for 'excess nourishment', hypertrophy is an increase in the volume of a muscle or organ caused by enlargement of its cells.

ISOLATION LIFT

An exercise involving movement in only one joint, such as the biceps curl (elbow) and leg extension (knee). They're great at the end of a workout when you can work a muscle to failure.

MUSCLE PUMP

When your muscles are engorged with blood after you've repeatedly shortened and lengthened it. Typically this occurs after weight training but can be achieved by repeatedly flexing your muscles.

REPS

Abbreviation of repetition. One rep is the completion of a given exercise from start to finish through a full range of motion. The number of reps per set can vary from one to more than 20, depending on your goals.

REST INTERVAL

The time you take between exercises and/or sets, during which your muscles can replenish their energy stores. The amount of rest can be manipulated depending on your training goals.

SETS

A given number of reps of a single exercise performed consecutively without rest. The number of sets performed of each exercise can vary depending on the workout.

SUPERCOMPENSATION

The period after training and recovery when you're fitter and stronger than before. Training in this window will result in further gains in strength, size and fitness. Training before this window, on the other hand, can result in overtraining, while training after it has closed reduces your ability to make additional gains.

TEMPO

The speed at which you perform a lift. Tempo is detailed by a four-digit code, such as 4010. The first number is the time in seconds the weight is lowered; the second is the time in seconds the move is held at the bottom position; the third is the time in seconds that the weight it lifted (if 'X' is shown this means lift explosively); and the final digit is the time in seconds the weight is held at the top of the move.

Men's Fitness

Helping you get fit and stay fit – wherever you are

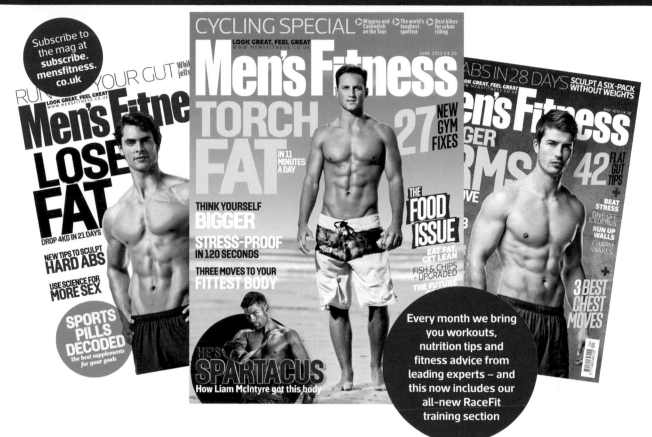

Subscribe to the mag at subscribe. mensfitness.co.uk

Every month we bring you workouts, nutrition tips and fitness advice from leading experts – and this now includes our all-new RaceFit training section

---

▷ New! Interactive iPad issue

The interactive edition of *Men's Fitness* includes exclusive videos to help you get the most from your workouts, plus all the expert advice that makes *MF* such an essential training tool

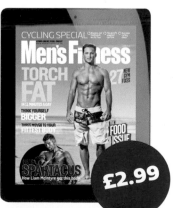

£2.99

Available on the App Store

▷ New! Visit the *MF* shop

Want the best fitness equipment from leading brands at great prices? Then pay a visit to the *MF* shop at shop.mensfitness.co.uk

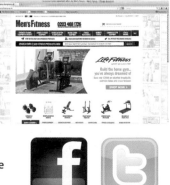

▷ Find us at
f MensFitnessMagazine
t @MensFitnessMag

---

www.mensfitness.co.uk

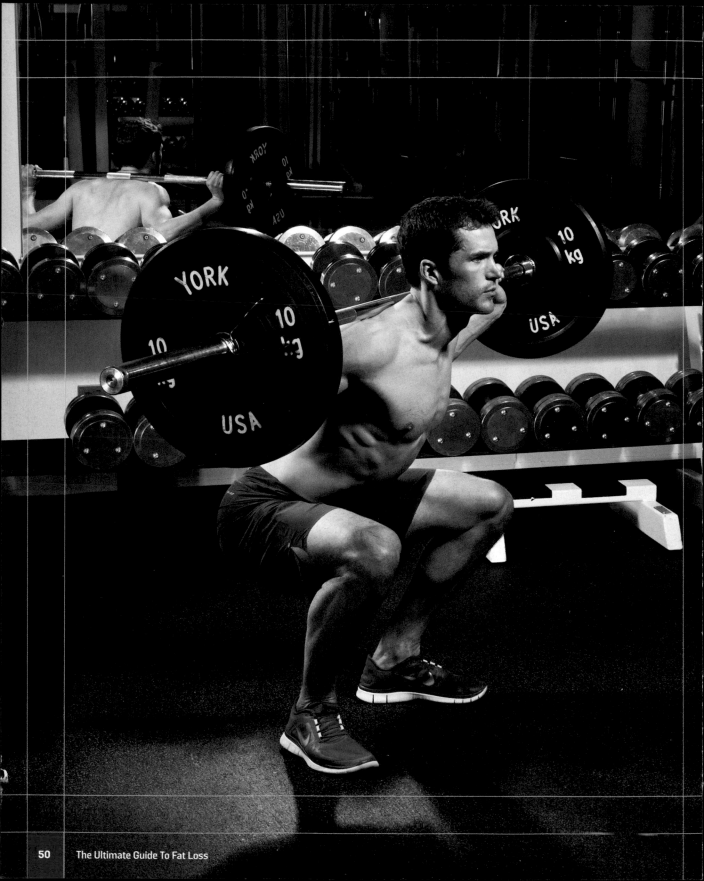

BURN, BABY, BURN

Turn the page to begin your
six-week fat-loss journey

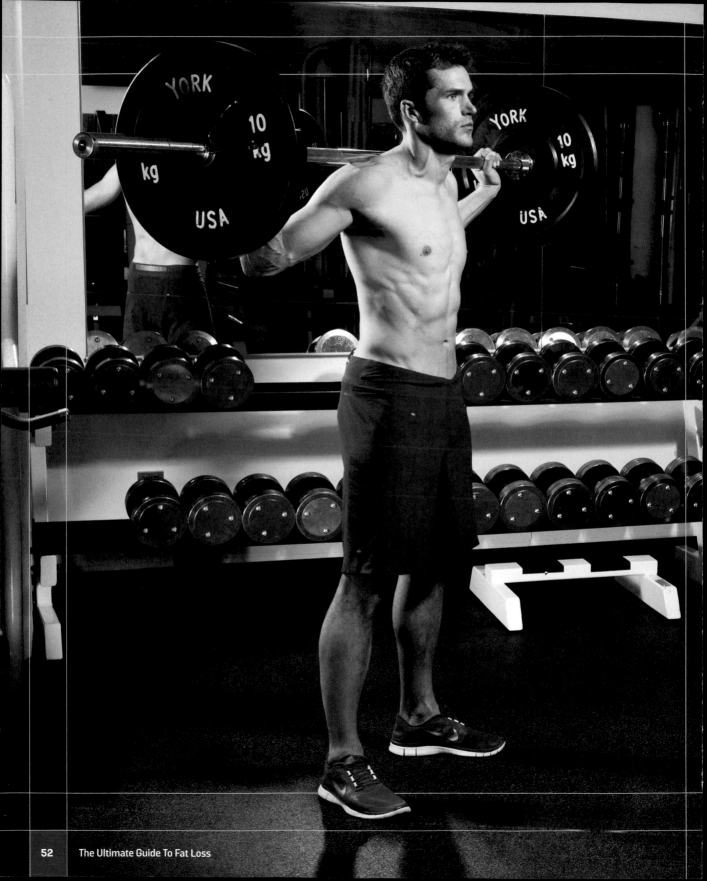

WEEK ONE

Turn the page for the **first week** of your **six-week** nutrition and exercise plan

THIS WEEK'S MENU

MONDAY	TUESDAY	WEDNESDAY	THURSDAY
BREAKFAST ■ Beef slices, ½ avocado and asparagus	**BREAKFAST** ■ Roast chicken slices, spinach and a handful of mixed nuts	**BREAKFAST** ■ Two scrambled eggs with smoked salmon, steamed kale and ½ avocado	**BREAKFAST** ■ Spinach and goat's cheese omelette with a handful of almonds
SNACK ■ Post-workout shake: blend 1 scoop protein powder, 230ml coconut milk, 1tsp almond butter, ½ banana and ice	**SNACK** ■ 50g cottage cheese with celery, carrot and cucumber sticks	**SNACK** ■ Post-workout shake: blend 1 scoop protein powder, 230ml coconut milk, 1tsp almond butter, a handful of blueberries and ice	**SNACK** ■ Small pot of hummus with sugar snap peas, carrots and celery
LUNCH ■ 100g quinoa mixed with 1 chopped onion, crushed garlic, 1 chopped green chilli and 8 walnuts, served with 1 salmon fillet	**LUNCH** ■ Ham salad with ½ avocado	**LUNCH** ■ Smoked salmon with spinach, cucumber and mixed salad leaves	**LUNCH** ■ Roast chicken with baked sweet potato and runner beans
SNACK ■ Guacamole made with ¼ tomato, lime juice, ¼ red onion, coriander and ½ ripe avocado, served with sugar snap peas	**SNACK** ■ 100g cooked prawns	**SNACK** ■ Guacamole made with ¼ tomato, lime juice, ¼ red onion, coriander and ½ ripe avocado, served with red pepper slices	**SNACK** ■ 100g cooked prawns
DINNER ■ Chicken and cashew nut stir-fry	**DINNER** ■ 1 cod fillet and roasted vegetables	**DINNER** ■ 1 salmon fillet with green beans and asparagus	**DINNER** ■ 2 homemade hamburgers with a spinach and cherry tomato salad
SNACK ■ Greek yoghurt with cinnamon and 8 macadamia nuts	**SNACK** ■ Greek yoghurt with cinnamon and 10 almonds	**SNACK** ■ Whey protein mixed with 1tbsp Greek yoghurt, water and ice	**SNACK** ■ Greek yoghurt with cinnamon and 10 almonds

Here's what you need to eat and when over the next seven days to blast away body fat

FRIDAY

BREAKFAST
- Beef slices, ½ avocado and asparagus

SNACK
- Post-workout shake: blend 1 scoop protein powder, 230ml coconut milk, 1tsp almond butter, ½ banana and ice

LUNCH
- Tuna salad

SNACK
- Guacamole made with ¼ tomato, lime juice, ¼ red onion, coriander and ½ ripe avocado, served with sugar snap peas

DINNER
- Grilled peppercorn ribeye steak and Dijon butter, served with steamed green vegetables

SNACK
- Greek yoghurt with cinnamon and 8 macadamia nuts

SATURDAY

BREAKFAST
- Bacon and 2 scrambled eggs

SNACK
- Small pot of hummus with celery, courgette and cucumber sticks

LUNCH
- Baked sweet potato with goat's cheese and spring onions, served with a side salad

SNACK
- 2 boiled eggs

DINNER
- Chicken stir-fry with beansprouts

SNACK
- Greek yoghurt with cinnamon and 10 almonds

SUNDAY

BREAKFAST
- 2 grilled venison sausages and 2 scrambled eggs

SNACK
- 50g cottage cheese with celery, carrot and cucumber sticks

LUNCH
- Diced lamb grilled on skewers with diced green and red peppers, cherry tomatoes and diced red onion, served with ½ baked sweet potato

SNACK
- 1 can salmon

DINNER
- 1 grilled salmon fillet with roasted vegetables

SNACK
- Greek yoghurt with cinnamon and 8 macadamia nuts

SHAKE IT!
Protein shakes have been included on Monday, Wednesday and Friday because it's an effective way to plan your gym workouts. If you train on other days, have shakes after those sessions instead.

WORKOUTS

Do the three workouts for this first week in order, leaving at least one day's rest between each one. A good approach would be to train on Monday, Wednesday and Friday, and do the high-intensity cardio session (see p70) over the weekend.

WEEK ONE UPPER BODY

		EXERCISE	SETS	REPS	TEMPO	REST
WORKOUT 1	1A	Dumbbell bench press	3	12	2010	10sec
	1B	Dumbbell shoulder press	3	12	2010	10sec
	1C	Dumbbell flye	3	10	2010	10sec
	1D	Dumbbell biceps curl	3	10	2010	90sec
	2A	Dumbbell bent-over row	3	12	2110	10sec
	2B	Dumbbell bent-over flye	3	12	2010	10sec
	2C	Underhand lat pull-down	3	10	2110	10sec
	2D	Seated row	3	10	2010	90sec

•• Perform the first sets of 1A, 1B, 1C and 1D, taking 10 seconds' rest between each. Then rest for 90 seconds and repeat until all three sets are completed.

•• Perform the first sets of 2A, 2B, 2C and 2D, taking 10 seconds' rest between each. Then rest for 90 seconds and repeat until all three sets are completed.

WEEK ONE ▸ LOWER BODY

		EXERCISE	SETS	REPS	TEMPO	REST
WORKOUT 2	1A	Dumbbell squat	3	12	2010	10sec
	1B	Dumbbell lunge	3	12	2010	10sec
	1C	Dumbbell side step-up	3	10	1010	10sec
	1D	Dumbbell step-up	3	10	1010	90sec
	2A	Bodyweight squat	3	12	2010	10sec
	2B	Bodyweight lunge	3	12	2010	10sec
	2C	Box jump	3	10	X	10sec
	2D	Tuck jump	3	10	X	90sec

•• Perform the first sets of 1A, 1B, 1C and 1D, taking 10 seconds' rest between each. Then rest for 90 seconds and repeat until all three sets are completed.

•• Perform the first sets of 2A, 2B, 2C and 2D, taking 10 seconds' rest between each. Then rest for 90 seconds and repeat until all three sets are completed.

WEEK ONE ▸ TOTAL BODY

		EXERCISE	SETS	REPS	TEMPO	REST
WORKOUT 3	1A	Deadlift	3	10	1111	10sec
	1B	Barbell bent-over row	3	10	1111	10sec
	1C	Shoulder press	3	10	3010	10sec
	1D	Squat	3	10	3010	90sec
	2A	Dumbbell squat to curl	3	12	1111	0sec
	2B	Dumbbell lunge to press	3	12	1111	0sec
	2C	Press-up	3	12	2010	0sec
	2D	Crunch	3	12	2110	90sec

•• Perform the first sets of 1A, 1B, 1C and 1D, taking 10 seconds' rest between each. Then rest for 90 seconds and repeat until all three sets are completed.

•• Perform the first sets of 2A, 2B, 2C and 2D without taking any rest between each. Then rest for 90 seconds and repeat until all three sets are completed.

1A Dumbbell bench press

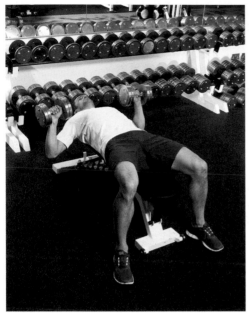
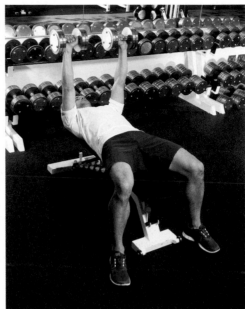

- Lie on a flat bench holding a dumbbell in each hand at shoulder height.
- Keep your feet flat on the floor and your upper back against the bench.
- Press the weights directly above your head but don't lock out your elbows at the top.
- Slowly lower the weights back to the start, flaring your elbows out to the sides as you do so.

1B Dumbbell shoulder press

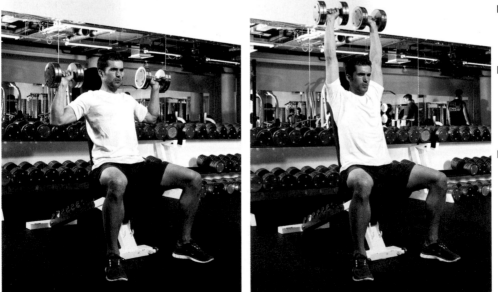

- Sit on an upright bench with your feet shoulder-width apart, holding a dumbbell in each hand at shoulder height.
- Keeping your chest upright and your core muscles braced, press the weights directly upwards until your arms are fully extended overhead.
- Lower the weights back to the start.

1C Dumbbell flye

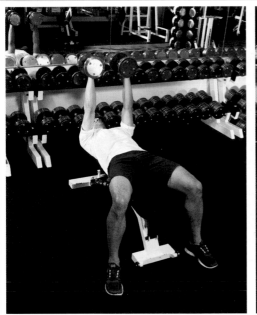 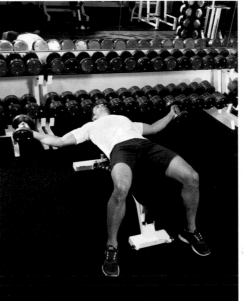

- Lie on a flat bench holding a dumbbell in each hand above your chest with your palms facing.
- Keep your feet flat on the floor and your upper back against the bench.
- With a slight bend in your elbows, lower the weights out to the sides as far as is comfortable.
- Use your chest muscles to reverse the movement and raise the weights back to the start.

1D Dumbbell biceps curl

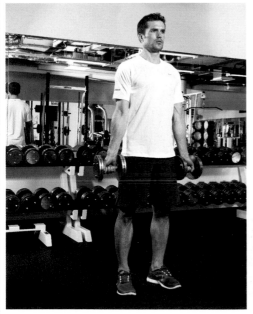 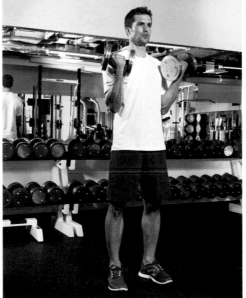

- Stand tall, holding a dumbbell in each hand by your sides with your palms facing forwards.
- Keeping your elbows tucked in, slowly raise both weights to shoulder height.
- At the top of the move squeeze your biceps and return slowly to the start.

2A Dumbbell bent-over row

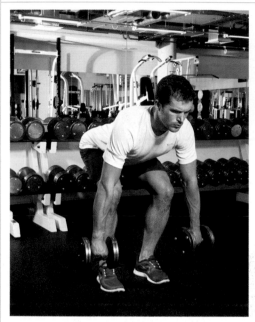
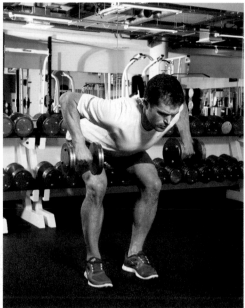

- Start with your core braced, your back straight and your shoulder blades retracted, holding a dumbbell in each hand with an overhand grip.
- Bend your knees slightly and lean forwards from the hips.
- Row the weights up to your lower sternum by retracting your shoulder blades, then slowly lower them again.

2B Dumbbell bent-over flye

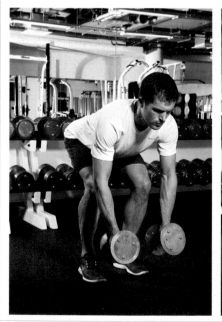
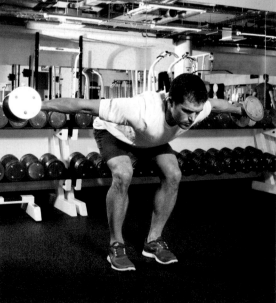

- Start with your core braced, your back straight and your shoulder blades retracted, holding a dumbbell in each hand with an overhand grip.
- Bend your knees slightly and lean forwards from the hips.
- With a slight bend in your elbows, raise the weights to the sides until they reach shoulder height, then slowly lower them again.

2C Underhand lat pull-down

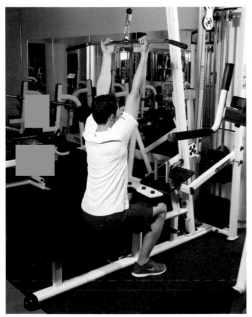 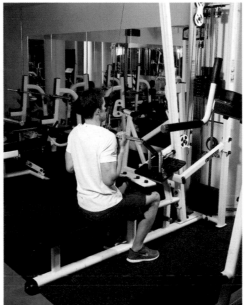

- Sit on the seat and take a narrow underhand grip on the bar.
- Look forwards, retract your shoulder blades and keep your torso upright.
- Pull the bar down in front of you until it reaches your upper chest. Don't lean back to aid the movement.
- At the bottom of the move squeeze your biceps and return slowly to the start.

2D Seated row

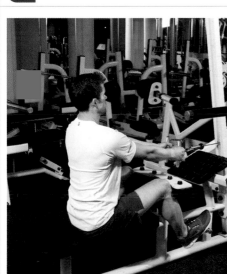 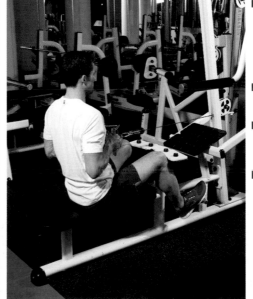

- Sit on the bench with a slight bend in your knees, holding a double-D handle with a neutral grip attached to the lower pulley of a cable machine.
- Ensure there's tension in the cable before you begin.
- Pull the handle into your sternum, keeping upper-body movement to a minimum.
- At the bottom of the move squeeze your shoulder blades together and return slowly to the start.

FAT-LOSS FINISHER
Burpee
p172

1A Dumbbell squat

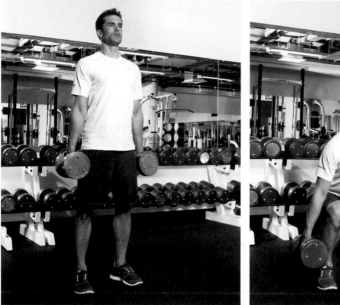
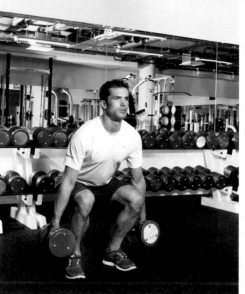

- Stand tall with your feet shoulder-width apart, holding a dumbbell in each hand by your sides.
- With your core braced and keeping a natural arch in your back, squat until your thighs are at least parallel to the floor, keeping your knees in line with your toes.
- Push back up through your heels to return to the start.

1B Dumbbell lunge

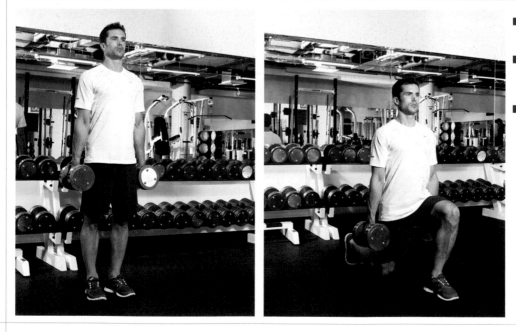

- Stand tall, holding a dumbbell in each hand by your sides.
- Take a big step forwards with one leg and lunge until both knees are bent at 90°.
- Push back off your front foot to return to the start, then repeat with the other leg. That's one rep.

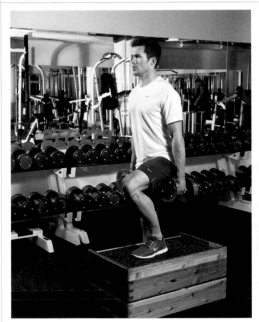
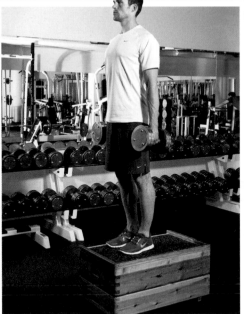

■ Stand side-on to a platform set at knee height, holding a dumbbell in each hand. Place one foot on the platform.

■ Keeping that foot on the platform, step up and back down with the other. That's one rep.

■ Complete the required number of reps with that foot, then swap feet and repeat.

1D Dumbbell step-up

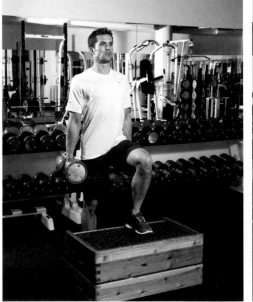
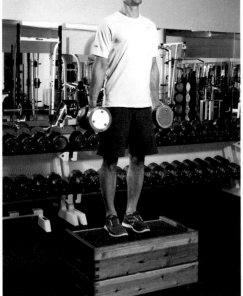

■ Stand side-on to a platform set at knee height, holding a dumbbell in each hand. Place one foot on the platform.

■ Keeping that foot on the platform, step up and back down with the other. That's one rep.

■ Complete the required number of reps with that foot, then swap feet and repeat.

2A Bodyweight squat

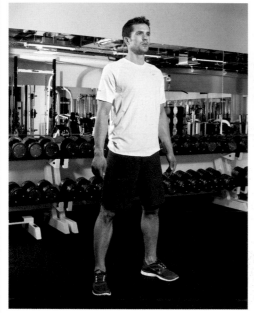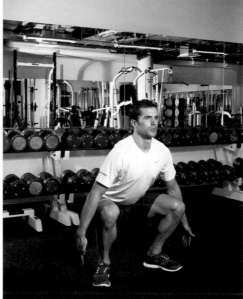

- Stand tall with your feet shoulder-width apart.
- With your core braced and keeping a natural arch in your back, squat until your thighs are at least parallel to the floor, keeping your knees in line with your toes.
- Push back up through your heels to return to the start.

2B Bodyweight lunge

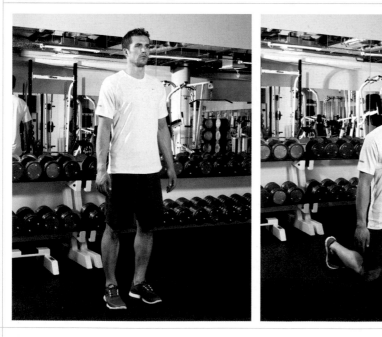

- Stand tall. Take a big step forwards with one leg and lunge until both knees are bent at 90°.
- Push back off your front foot to return to the start, then repeat with the other leg. That's one rep.

2C Box jump

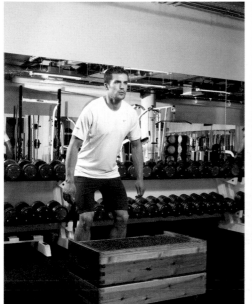
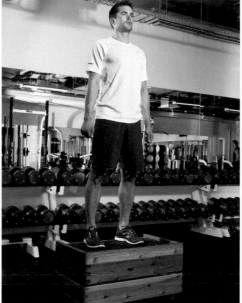

- Stand in front of a box or raised platform.
- Explosively jump on to the box, landing with both feet.
- Step back down to return to the start.

2D Tuck jump

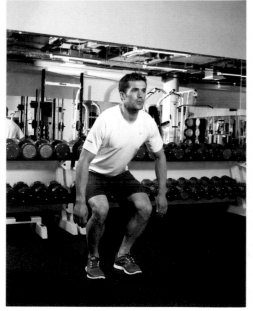
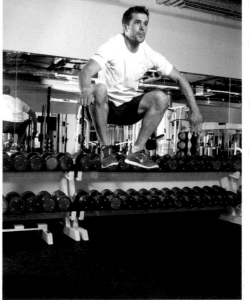

- Stand tall with your feet shoulder-width apart and your core braced.
- Squat until your thighs are at least parallel to the floor, keeping your knees in line with your toes.
- Jump off the ground explosively, pulling your knees towards your chest.
- As you land descend straight into the next rep.

FAT-LOSS FINISHER
Kettlebell swing
p173

1A Deadlift

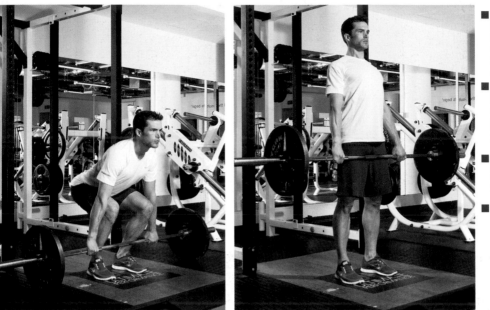

- Stand in front of a barbell. Squat and take hold of the bar with an overhand or alternate grip just outside your knees.
- Keeping your core braced and your shoulders back, use your glutes to power the initial lift, pushing down through your heels.
- Keep the bar close to your body and as the bar passes your knees push your hips forwards.
- Reverse the move to return to the start.

1B Barbell bent-over row

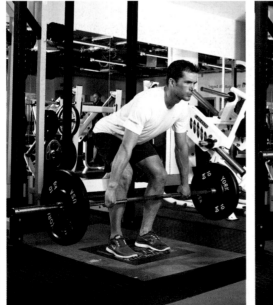

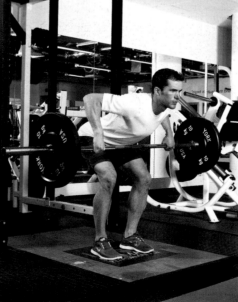

- With your core braced, your back straight and your shoulders back, bend your knees slightly and lean forwards from your hips.
- Grip the barbell with your hands slightly more than shoulder-width apart, letting it hang at knee level.
- Pull the bar up to your lower sternum, retracting your shoulder blades. Lower the bar slowly.

1C Shoulder press

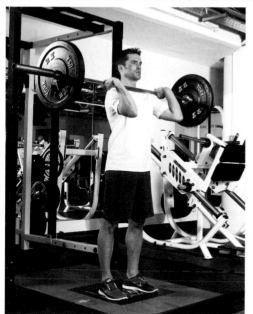 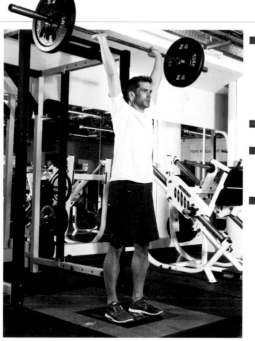

- Stand tall with your feet shoulder-width apart. Rest the barbell on your upper chest, holding it with your hands slightly more than shoulder-width apart.
- Keep your chest upright and your core braced.
- Press the bar directly upwards until your arms are fully extended. Don't tilt your hips forwards.
- Lower the bar to return to the start.

1D Squat

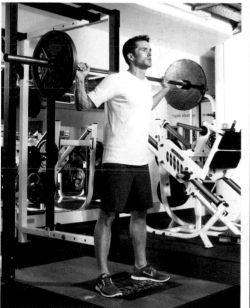 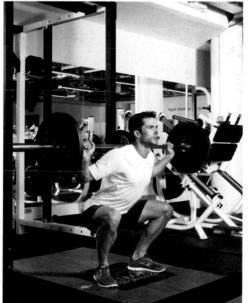

- Rest a barbell on the back of your shoulders – not your neck – holding it with an overhand grip slightly wider than your shoulders. Keep your elbows pointing to the floor.
- Your feet should be slightly more than shoulder-width apart with your toes pointing outwards slightly.
- Squat until your thighs are at least parallel to the floor, keeping your knees in line with your toes.
- Push back up through your heels to return to the start.

2A Dumbbell squat to curl

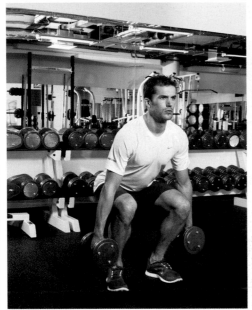
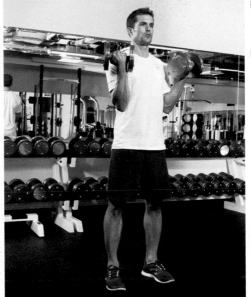

- Stand tall with your feet shoulder-width apart, holding a dumbbell in each hand by your sides.
- With your core braced and keeping a natural arch in your back, squat until your thighs are at least parallel to the floor, keeping your knees in line with your toes.
- Push back up through your heels to stand. Keeping your elbows by your sides, curl the weights up to your shoulders.
- Lower the weights and descend straight into the next rep.

2B Dumbbell lunge to press

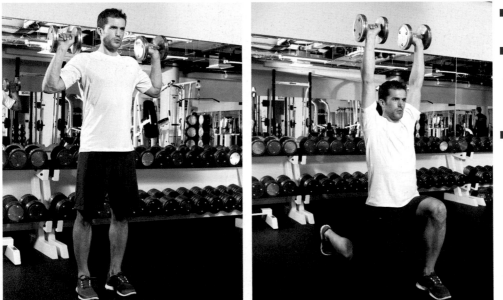

- Stand tall, holding a dumbbell in each hand at shoulder height.
- Take a big step forwards with one leg and lunge until both knees are bent at 90°. At the same time, press the weights directly above your head.
- Push back off your front foot to return to standing, while lowering the weights. Repeat with the other leg. That's one rep.

2C Press-up

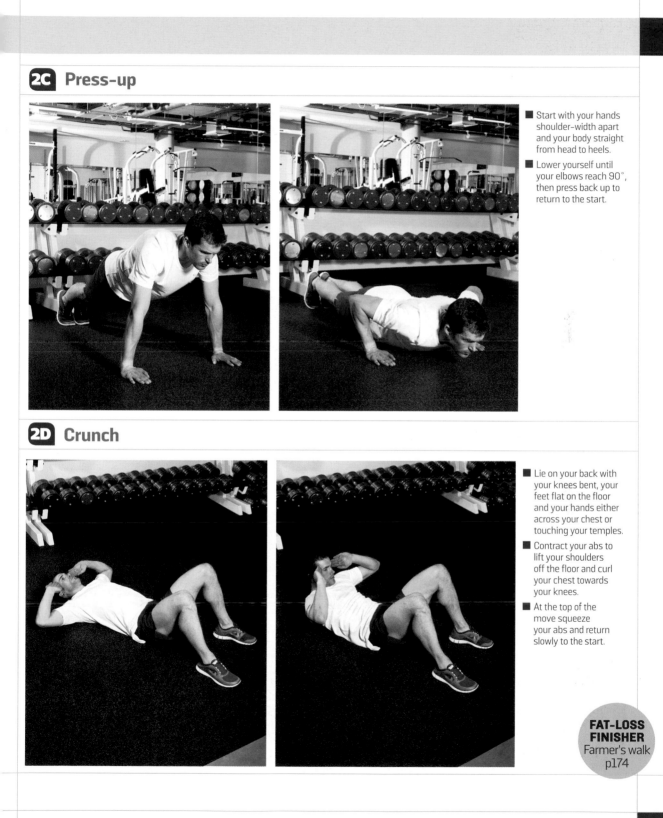

- Start with your hands shoulder-width apart and your body straight from head to heels.
- Lower yourself until your elbows reach 90°, then press back up to return to the start.

2D Crunch

- Lie on your back with your knees bent, your feet flat on the floor and your hands either across your chest or touching your temples.
- Contract your abs to lift your shoulders off the floor and curl your chest towards your knees.
- At the top of the move squeeze your abs and return slowly to the start.

FAT-LOSS FINISHER
Farmer's walk
p174

GET MOVING

Choose your activity to complete this week's training programme

The fourth and final session of week one is a 25-minute high-intensity cardio session. Whether you run, cycle or row is up to you. To complete the session, simply follow the charts below to make sure you work your muscles and cardiovascular system to burn the optimum amount of body fat.

🏃 RUN		🚴 BIKE		🚣 ROW	
DURATION	INTENSITY	DURATION	INTENSITY	DURATION	INTENSITY
5min	2	5min	2	5min	2
5min	3	5min	3	5min	3
30sec	4	30sec	4	30sec	4
1min	3	1min	3	1min	3
30sec	4	30sec	4	30sec	4
1min	3	1min	3	1min	3
30sec	4	30sec	4	30sec	4
45sec	3	45sec	3	45sec	3
45sec	4	45sec	4	45sec	4
30sec	3	30sec	3	30sec	3
45sec	4	45sec	4	45sec	4
15sec	5	15sec	5	15sec	5
1min	2	1min	2	1min	2
45sec	4	45sec	4	45sec	4
15sec	5	15sec	5	15sec	5
30sec	3	30sec	3	30sec	3
45sec	4	45sec	4	45sec	4
15sec	5	15sec	5	15sec	5
3min	3	3min	3	3min	3
1min	2	1min	2	1min	2
1min	1	1min	1	1min	1

HOW HARD SHOULD YOU WORK?

Use this key to discover how much effort you should put in during every interval

1 Easy	2 Comfortable	3 Moderate	4 Intense	5 All-out

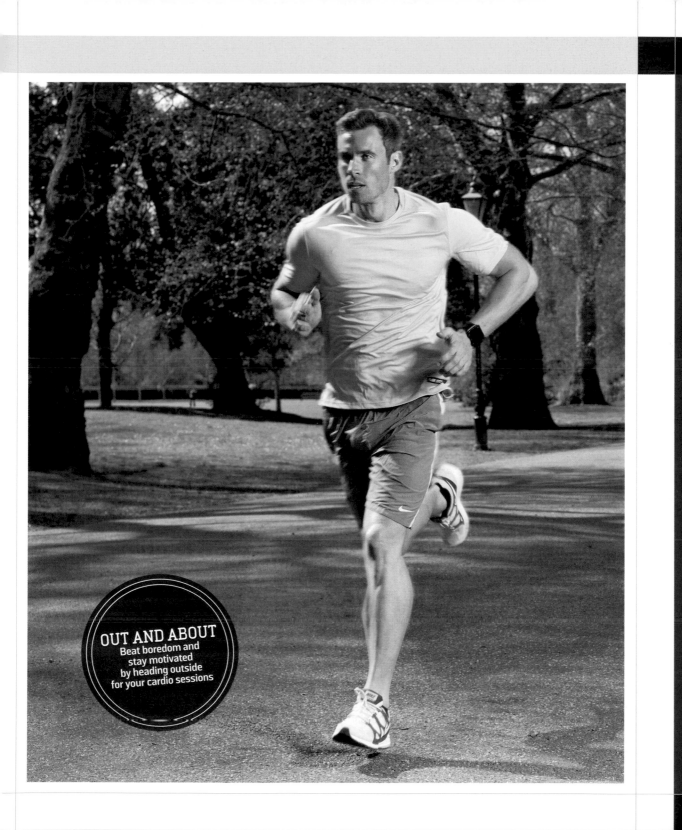

OUT AND ABOUT
Beat boredom and
stay motivated
by heading outside
for your cardio sessions

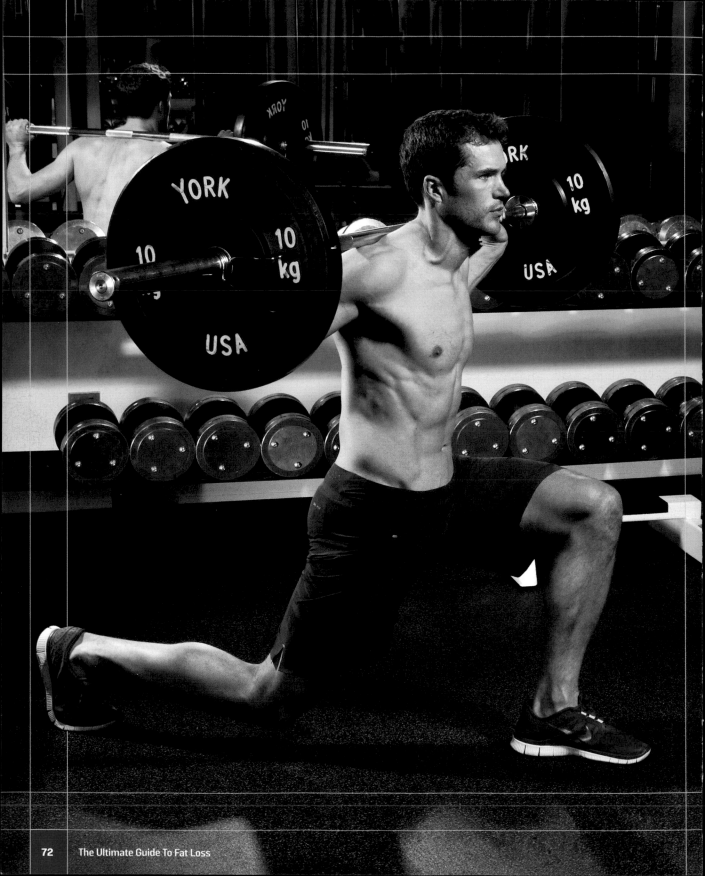

WEEK TWO

Turn the page for the **second week** of your **six-week** nutrition and exercise plan

THIS WEEK'S MENU

MONDAY	TUESDAY	WEDNESDAY	THURSDAY
BREAKFAST ■ Roast chicken slices, spinach and a handful of mixed nuts	**BREAKFAST** ■ Beef slices, ½ avocado and asparagus	**BREAKFAST** ■ 3-egg omelette with mixed peppers	**BREAKFAST** ■ Roast chicken slices, spinach and a handful of mixed nuts
SNACK ■ Post-workout shake: blend 1 scoop protein powder, 200ml almond milk, 1tsp brazil nut butter and 1tbsp flax seeds	**SNACK** ■ 2 boiled eggs	**SNACK** ■ Post-workout shake: blend 1 scoop protein powder, 200ml almond milk, 1tsp brazil nut butter and 1tbsp flax seeds	**SNACK** ■ Ham and ½ avocado
LUNCH ■ Grilled prawns with salad, avocado and pumpkin seeds	**LUNCH** ■ Chicken stir-fry	**LUNCH** ■ 2 homemade hamburgers with spinach salad, cherry tomatoes and chopped onion	**LUNCH** ■ Tuna salad, served with 1 baked sweet potato
SNACK ■ 2 boiled eggs	**SNACK** ■ Guacamole and raw vegetables	**SNACK** ■ Guacamole and sliced red pepper	**SNACK** ■ Greek yoghurt
DINNER ■ Beef meatballs in tomato sauce, with spinach and green vegetables	**DINNER** ■ Chicken wrapped in Parma ham, with sweet potato mash and broccoli	**DINNER** ■ 2 grilled turkey breasts, with broccoli and mange tout	**DINNER** ■ Steak with roasted vegetables
SNACK ■ Greek yoghurt with cinnamon and 6 brazil nuts	**SNACK** ■ Greek yoghurt with cinnamon and 10 almonds	**SNACK** ■ Greek yoghurt with cinnamon and 6 brazil nuts	**SNACK** ■ 50g cottage cheese with ½ punnet blueberries and 1tbsp pumpkin seeds

Here's what you need to eat and when over the next seven days to blast away body fat

FRIDAY	SATURDAY	SUNDAY

BREAKFAST
- 2 poached eggs, smoked salmon and ½ avocado

SNACK
- Post-workout shake: blend 1 scoop protein powder, 200ml almond milk, 1tsp brazil nut butter and 1tbsp flax seeds

LUNCH
- Grilled prawns with salad, avocado and pumpkin seeds

SNACK
- Guacamole and sliced red pepper

DINNER
- 1 cod fillet with asparagus and green beans; 1 small glass red wine

SNACK
- Greek yoghurt with cinnamon and 6 brazil nuts

BREAKFAST
- 2 scrambled eggs, ½ can cooked tomatoes, ½ can reduced salt and sugar beans, mushrooms and 2 rashers grilled bacon

SNACK
- 1tbsp brazil nut butter and cucumber slices

LUNCH
- Chicken stir-fry

SNACK
- 1 can tuna

DINNER
- 2 homemade hamburgers with spinach salad, cherry tomatoes and chopped onion

SNACK
- Whey protein mixed with 1tbsp Greek yoghurt, water and ice

BREAKFAST
- 2 scrambled eggs, ½ can cooked tomatoes, ½ can of reduced salt and sugar beans, mushrooms and 2 rashers grilled bacon

SNACK
- Smoked salmon and ½ avocado

LUNCH
- Beef stir-fry

SNACK
- 1tbsp brazil nut butter and cucumber slices

DINNER
- 2 grilled turkey breasts, with broccoli and asparagus

SNACK
- Whey protein mixed with 1tbsp Greek yoghurt, water and ice

SHAKE IT!
Protein shakes have been included on Monday, Wednesday and Friday because it's an effective way to plan your gym workouts. If you train on other days, have shakes after those sessions instead.

WORKOUTS

Do the three workouts for the second week in order, leaving at least one day's rest between each one. If possible, train on the same days as in week one and don't forget to leave time for the high-intensity cardio session (see p90).

WEEK TWO   UPPER BODY

		EXERCISE	SETS	REPS	TEMPO	REST
WORKOUT 1	1A	Dumbbell bench press	4	10	2010	10sec
	1B	Dumbbell shoulder press	4	10	2010	10sec
	1C	Dumbbell flye	4	8	2010	10sec
	1D	Dumbbell biceps curl	4	8	2010	90sec
	2A	Dumbbell bent-over row	4	10	2110	10sec
	2B	Dumbbell bent-over flye	4	10	2010	10sec
	2C	Underhand lat pull-down	4	8	2110	10sec
	2D	Seated row	4	8	2110	90sec

•• Perform the first sets of 1A, 1B, 1C and 1D, taking 10 seconds' rest between each. Then rest for 90 seconds and repeat until all four sets are completed.

•• Perform the first sets of 2A, 2B, 2C and 2D, taking 10 seconds' rest between each. Then rest for 90 seconds and repeat until all four sets are completed.

WEEK TWO   LOWER BODY

WORKOUT 2

	EXERCISE	SETS	REPS	TEMPO	REST
1A	Dumbbell squat	4	10	2010	10sec
1B	Dumbbell lunge	4	10	2010	10sec
1C	Dumbbell side step-up	4	8	1010	10sec
1D	Dumbbell step-up	4	8	1010	90sec
2A	Bodyweight squat	4	10	2010	10sec
2B	Bodyweight lunge	4	10	2010	10sec
2C	Box jump	4	8	X	10sec
2D	Tuck jump	4	8	X	90sec

●● Perform the first sets of 1A, 1B, 1C and 1D, taking 10 seconds' rest between each. Then rest for 90 seconds and repeat until all four sets are completed.

●● Perform the first sets of 2A, 2B, 2C and 2D, taking 10 seconds' rest between each. Then rest for 90 seconds and repeat until all four sets are completed.

WEEK TWO   TOTAL BODY

WORKOUT 3

	EXERCISE	SETS	REPS	TEMPO	REST
1A	Deadlift	4	8	1111	10sec
1B	Barbell bent-over row	4	8	1111	10sec
1C	Shoulder press	4	8	3010	10sec
1D	Squat	4	8	3010	90sec
2A	Dumbbell squat to curl	4	10	1111	0sec
2B	Dumbbell lunge to press	4	10	1111	0sec
2C	Press-up	4	10	2010	0sec
2D	Crunch	4	10	2110	90sec

●● Perform the first sets of 1A, 1B, 1C and 1D, taking 10 seconds' rest between each. Then rest for 90 seconds and repeat until all four sets are completed.

●● Perform the first sets of 2A, 2B, 2C and 2D without taking any rest between each. Then rest for 90 seconds and repeat until all four sets are completed.

1A Dumbbell bench press

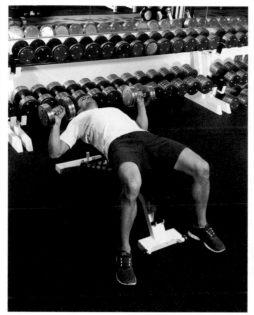 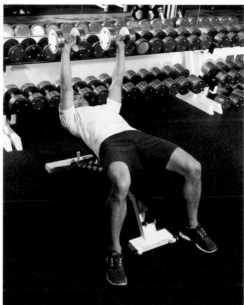

- Lie on a flat bench holding a dumbbell in each hand at shoulder height.
- Keep your feet flat on the floor and your upper back against the bench.
- Press the weights directly above your head but don't lock out your elbows at the top.
- Slowly lower the weights back to the start, flaring your elbows out to the sides as you do so.

1B Dumbbell shoulder press

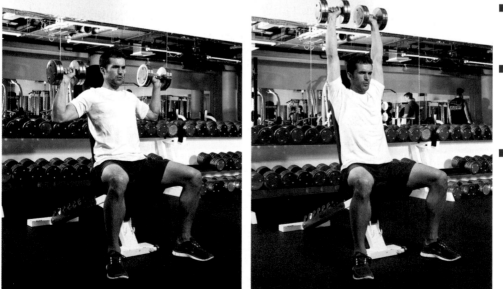

- Sit on an upright bench with your feet shoulder-width apart, holding a dumbbell in each hand at shoulder height.
- Keeping your chest upright and your core muscles braced, press the weights directly upwards until your arms are fully extended overhead.
- Lower the weights back to the start.

1C Dumbbell flye

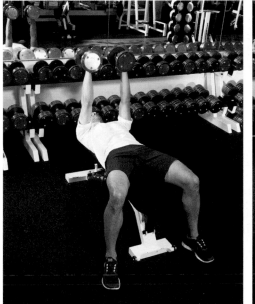
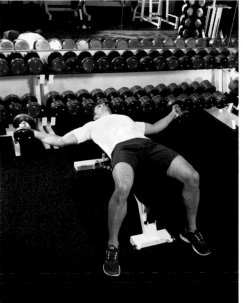

- Lie on a flat bench holding a dumbbell in each hand above your chest with your palms facing.
- Keep your feet flat on the floor and your upper back against the bench.
- With a slight bend in your elbows, lower the weights out to the sides as far as is comfortable.
- Use your chest muscles to reverse the movement and raise the weights back to the start.

1D Dumbbell biceps curl

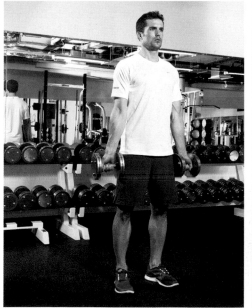
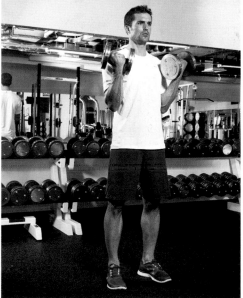

- Stand tall, holding a dumbbell in each hand by your sides with your palms facing forwards.
- Keeping your elbows tucked in, slowly raise both weights to shoulder height.
- At the top of the move squeeze your biceps and return slowly to the start.

2A Dumbbell bent-over row

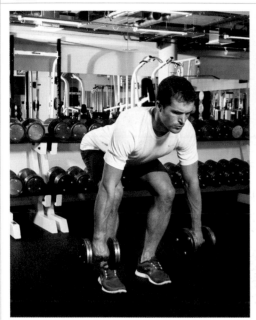
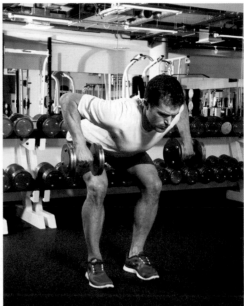

- Start with your core braced, your back straight and your shoulder blades retracted, holding a dumbbell in each hand with an overhand grip.
- Bend your knees slightly and lean forwards from the hips.
- Row the weights up to your lower sternum by retracting your shoulder blades, then slowly lower them again.

2B Dumbbell bent-over flye

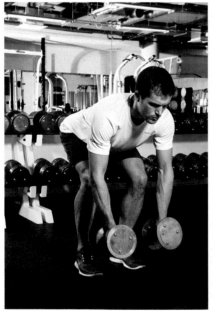
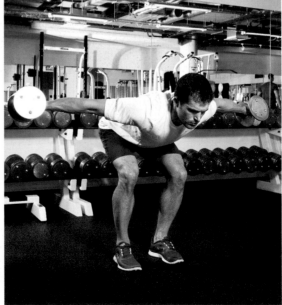

- Start with your core braced, your back straight and your shoulder blades retracted, holding a dumbbell in each hand with an overhand grip.
- Bend your knees slightly and lean forwards from the hips.
- With a slight bend in your elbows, raise the weights to the sides until they reach shoulder height, then slowly lower them again.

2C Underhand lat pull-down

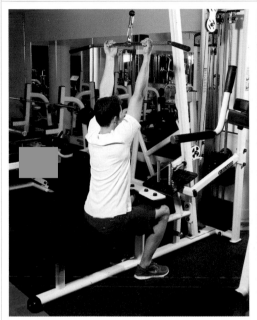
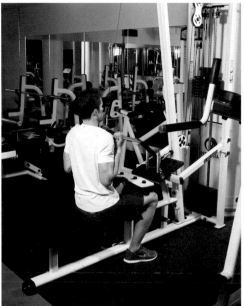

- Sit on the seat and take a narrow, underhand grip on the bar.
- Look forwards, retract your shoulder blades and keep your torso upright.
- Pull the bar down in front of you until it reaches your upper chest. Don't lean back to aid the movement.
- Squeeze your biceps at the bottom of the move and return the bar slowly to the start.

2D Seated row

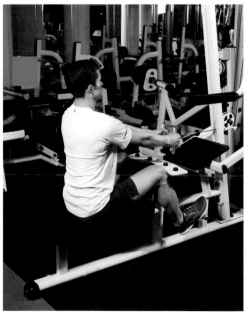
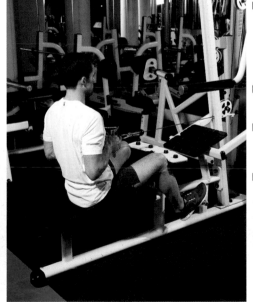

- Sit on the bench with a slight bend in your knees, holding a double-D handle with a neutral grip attached to the lower pulley of a cable machine.
- Ensure there's tension in the cable before you begin.
- Pull the handle into your sternum, keeping upper-body movement to a minimum.
- At the bottom of the move squeeze your shoulder blades together and return slowly to the start.

FAT-LOSS FINISHER Burpee p172

1A Dumbbell squat

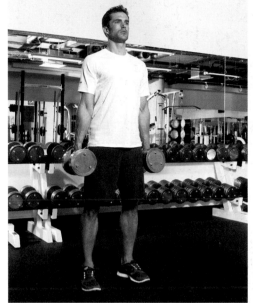
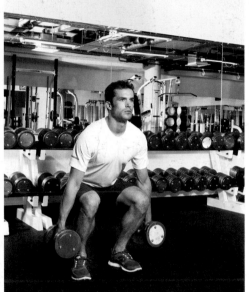

- Stand tall with your feet shoulder-width apart, holding a dumbbell in each hand by your sides.
- With your core braced and keeping a natural arch in your back, squat until your thighs are at least parallel to the floor, keeping your knees in line with your toes.
- Push back up through your heels to return to the start.

1B Dumbbell lunge

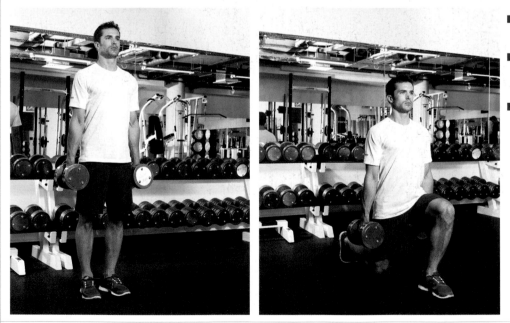

- Stand tall, holding a dumbbell in each hand by your sides.
- Take a big step forwards with one leg and lunge until both knees are bent at 90°.
- Push back off your front foot to return to the start, then repeat with the other leg. That's one rep.

1C Dumbbell side step-up

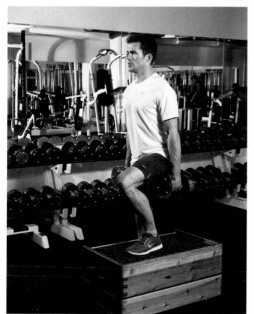
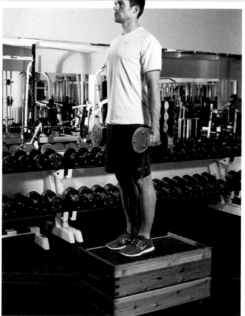

- Stand side-on to a platform set at knee height, holding a dumbbell in each hand. Place one foot on the platform.
- Keeping that foot on the platform, step up and back down with the other. That's one rep.
- Complete the required number of reps with that foot, then swap feet and repeat.

1D Dumbbell step-up

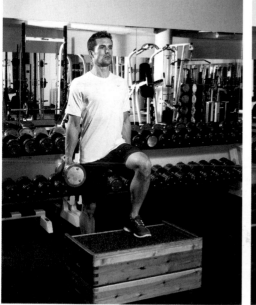
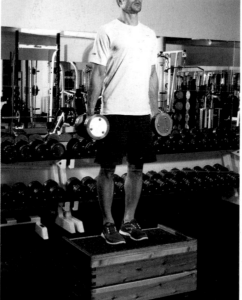

- Stand side-on to a platform set at knee height, holding a dumbbell in each hand. Place one foot on the platform.
- Keeping that foot on the platform, step up and back down with the other. That's one rep.
- Complete the required number of reps with that foot, then swap feet and repeat.

2A Bodyweight squat

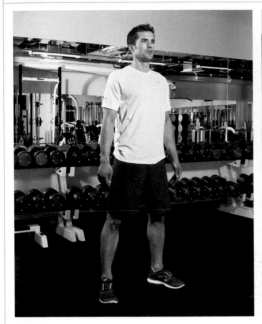
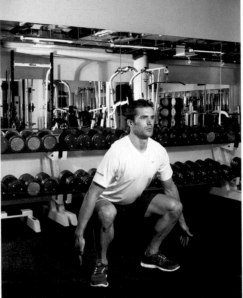

- Stand tall with your feet shoulder-width apart.
- With your core braced and keeping a natural arch in your back, squat until your thighs are at least parallel to the floor, keeping your knees in line with your toes.
- Push back up through your heels to return to the start.

2B Bodyweight lunge

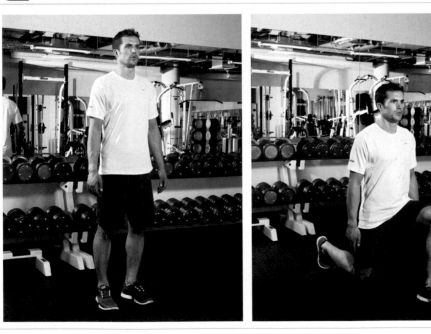

- Stand tall. Take a big step forwards with one leg and lunge until both knees are bent at 90°.
- Push back off your front foot to return to the start, then repeat with the other leg. That's one rep.

2C Box jump

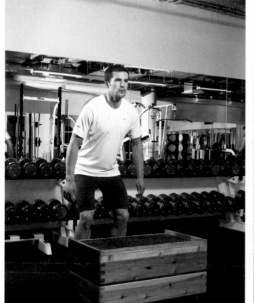

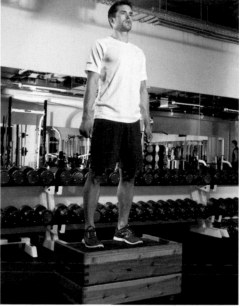

- Stand in front of a box or raised platform.
- Explosively jump on to the box, landing with both feet.
- Step back down to return to the start.

2D Tuck jump

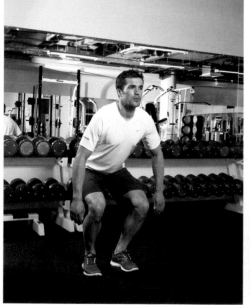

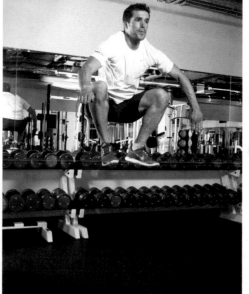

- Stand tall with your feet shoulder-width apart and your core braced.
- Squat until your thighs are at least parallel to the floor, keeping your knees in line with your toes.
- Jump off the ground explosively, pulling your knees towards your chest.
- As you land descend straight into the next rep.

FAT-LOSS FINISHER
Kettlebell swing
p173

1A Deadlift

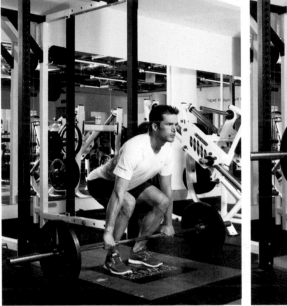
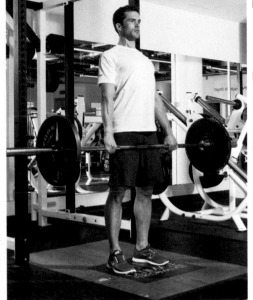

- Stand in front of a barbell. Squat and take hold of the bar with an overhand or alternate grip just outside your knees.
- Keeping your core braced and your shoulders back, use your glutes to power the initial lift, pushing down through your heels.
- Keep the bar close to your body and as the bar passes your knees push your hips forwards.
- Reverse the move to return to the start.

1B Barbell bent–over row

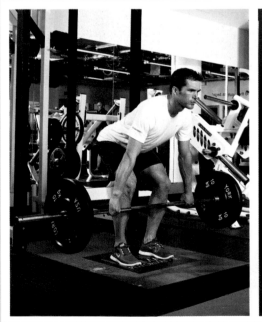
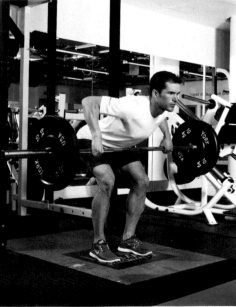

- With your core braced, your back straight and your shoulders back, bend your knees slightly and lean forwards from your hips.
- Grip the barbell with your hands slightly more than shoulder–width apart, letting it hang at knee level.
- Pull the bar up to your lower sternum, retracting your shoulder blades. Lower the bar slowly.

1C Shoulder press

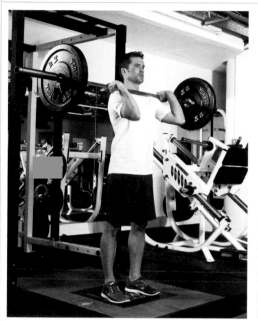

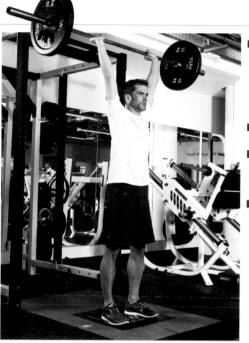

- Stand tall with your feet shoulder-width apart. Rest the barbell on your upper chest, holding it with your hands slightly more than shoulder-width apart.
- Keep your chest upright and your core braced.
- Press the bar directly upwards until your arms are fully extended. Don't tilt your hips forwards.
- Lower the bar to return to the start.

1D Squat

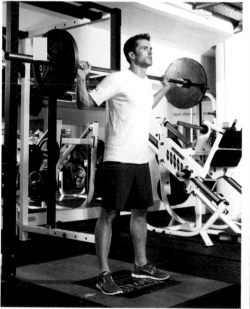

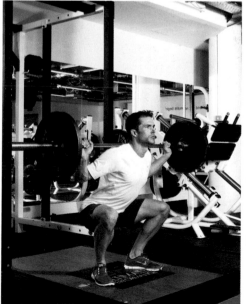

- Rest a barbell on the back of your shoulders – not your neck – holding it with an overhand grip slightly wider than your shoulders. Keep your elbows pointing to the floor.
- Your feet should be slightly more than shoulder-width apart with your toes pointing outwards slightly
- Squat until your thighs are at least parallel to the floor, keeping your knees in line with your toes.
- Push back up through your heels to return to the start.

2A Dumbbell squat to curl

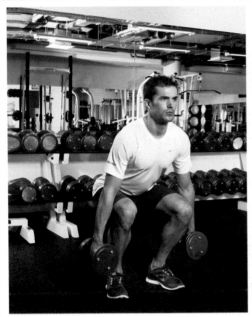
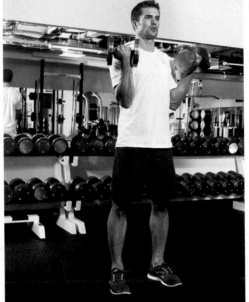

- Stand tall with your feet shoulder-width apart, holding a dumbbell in each hand by your sides.
- With your core braced and keeping a natural arch in your back, squat until your thighs are at least parallel to the floor, keeping your knees in line with your toes.
- Push back up through your heels to stand. Keeping your elbows by your sides, curl the weights up to your shoulders.
- Lower the weights and descend straight into the next rep.

2B Dumbbell lunge to press

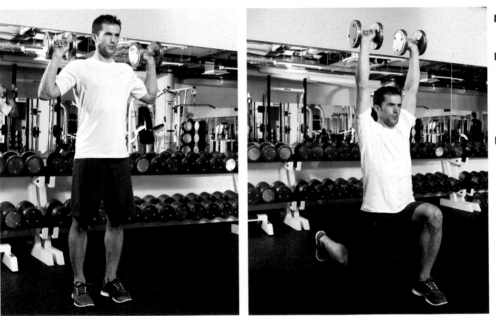

- Stand tall, holding a dumbbell in each hand at shoulder height.
- Take a big step forwards with one leg and lunge until both knees are bent at 90°. At the same time, press the weights directly above your head.
- Push back off your front foot to return to standing, while lowering the weights. Repeat with the other leg. That's one rep.

2C Press-up

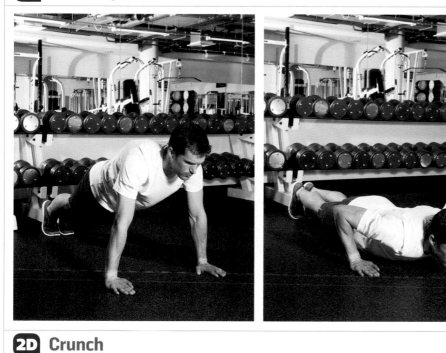

- Start with your hands shoulder-width apart and body straight from head to heels.
- Lower your chest down towards the floor until your elbows reach 90°, then press back up.

2D Crunch

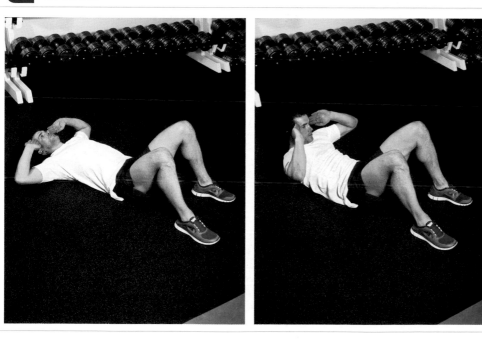

- Lie on your back with your knees bent, your feet flat on the floor and your hands either across your chest or touching your temples.
- Contract your abs to lift your shoulders off the floor and curl your chest towards your knees.
- At the top of the move squeeze your abs and return slowly to the start.

FAT-LOSS FINISHER
Farmer's walk
p174

GET MOVING

Choose your activity to complete this week's training programme

The fourth and final session of week one is a 25-minute high-intensity cardio session. Whether you run, cycle or row is up to you. To complete the session, simply follow the charts below to make sure you work your muscles and cardiovascular system to burn the optimum amount of body fat.

RUN DURATION	INTENSITY	BIKE DURATION	INTENSITY	ROW DURATION	INTENSITY
5min	2	5min	2	5min	2
5min	3	5min	3	5min	3
30sec	4	30sec	4	30sec	4
1min	3	1min	3	1min	3
30sec	4	30sec	4	30sec	4
1min	3	1min	3	1min	3
30sec	4	30sec	4	30sec	4
45sec	3	45sec	3	45sec	3
45sec	4	45sec	4	45sec	4
30sec	3	30sec	3	30sec	3
45sec	4	45sec	4	45sec	4
15sec	5	15sec	5	15sec	5
1min	2	1min	2	1min	2
45sec	4	45sec	4	45sec	4
15sec	5	15sec	5	15sec	5
30sec	3	30sec	3	30sec	3
45sec	4	45sec	4	45sec	4
15sec	5	15sec	5	15sec	5
3min	3	3min	3	3min	3
1min	2	1min	2	1min	2
1min	1	1min	1	1min	1

HOW HARD SHOULD YOU WORK?

Use this key to discover how much effort you should put in during every interval

1 Easy 2 Comfortable 3 Moderate 4 Intense 5 All-out

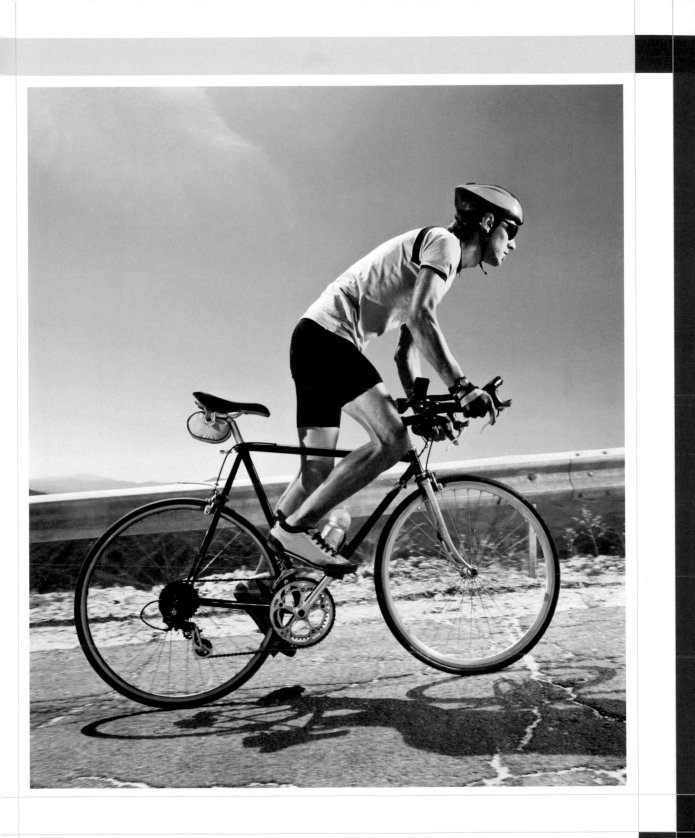

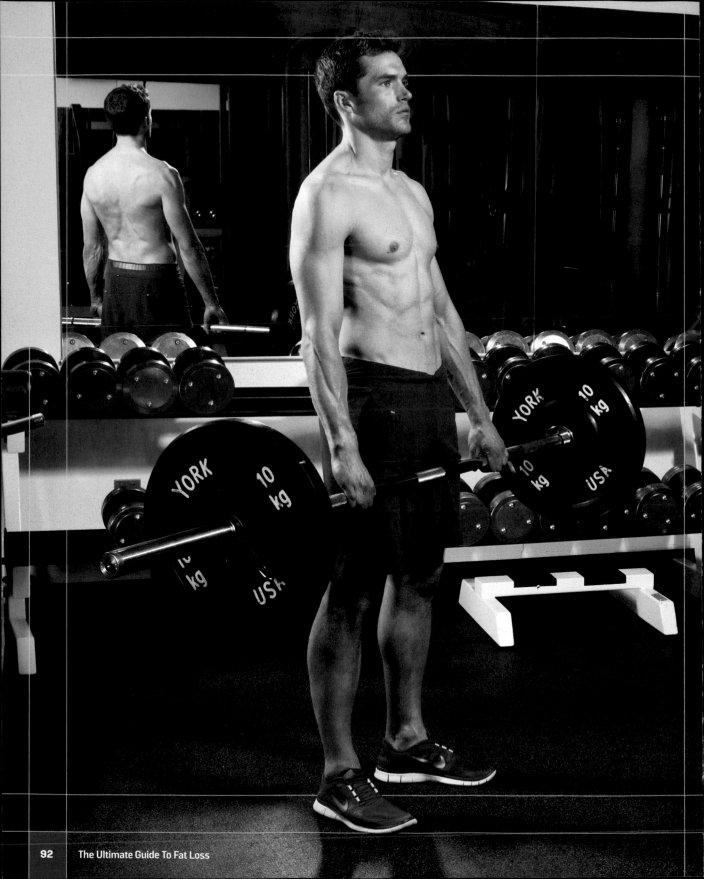

WEEK THREE

Turn the page for the **third week** of your **six-week** nutrition and exercise plan

THIS WEEK'S MENU

MONDAY	TUESDAY	WEDNESDAY	THURSDAY
BREAKFAST ◼ Roast chicken slices and roasted veg	**BREAKFAST** ◼ Beef slices, ½ avocado and asparagus	**BREAKFAST** ◼ 2 poached eggs, smoked salmon, steamed kale and ½ avocado	**BREAKFAST** ◼ Spinach and goat's cheese omelette and a handful of almonds
SNACK ◼ Post-workout shake: blend 1 scoop protein powder, 100ml almond milk, ½ banana, 75ml semi-skimmed milk and 1tbsp oats	**SNACK** ◼ Celery sticks, brazil nut butter and 10 raisins	**SNACK** ◼ Post-workout shake: blend 1 scoop protein powder, ½ banana, raspberries, 150ml skimmed milk, 100ml natural yoghurt, 1tbsp sunflower seeds and 20g rolled oats	**SNACK** ◼ Celery sticks and brazil nut butter
LUNCH ◼ 1 medium sweet potato with 1 can tuna in water (drained) and spinach	**LUNCH** ◼ Grilled prawns with a mixed salad, ½ avocado and pumpkin seeds	**LUNCH** ◼ Lamb steak with a side salad and cherry tomatoes	**LUNCH** ◼ Grilled prawns, mixed salad, ½ avocado and pumpkin seeds
SNACK ◼ Small pot of hummus with celery, carrot and cucumber sticks	**SNACK** ◼ 2 boiled eggs	**SNACK** ◼ Small pot of hummus with celery, carrot and cucumber sticks	**SNACK** ◼ 2 scrambled eggs, ham and spinach
DINNER ◼ Ginger chicken stir-fry	**DINNER** ◼ Chilli beef stuffed peppers and side salad	**DINNER** ◼ 1 cod fillet with steamed vegetables	**DINNER** ◼ Tuna steak, asparagus, broccoli and cauliflower
SNACK ◼ Greek yoghurt with cinnamon and pecan nuts	**SNACK** ◼ Greek yoghurt with cinnamon and 10 walnuts	**SNACK** ◼ Greek yoghurt with cinnamon and pecan nuts	**SNACK** ◼ Greek yoghurt with cinnamon and 10 walnuts

Here's what you need to eat and when over the next seven days to blast away body fat

FRIDAY	SATURDAY	SUNDAY

FRIDAY

BREAKFAST
- 150g porridge oats cooked with 200ml semi-skimmed milk, ½ banana and 1tsp honey; stir in ½ scoop whey protein at the end

SNACK
- Post-workout shake: blend 1 scoop protein powder, 100ml coconut milk, ½ banana, 75ml semi-skimmed milk and 1tbsp oats

LUNCH
- Ham and avocado salad

SNACK
- Small pot of hummus with celery, carrot and cucumber sticks

DINNER
- 2 pork chops with sweet potato mash and green beans; 1 small glass red wine

SNACK
- Greek yoghurt with cinnamon and pecan nuts

SATURDAY

BREAKFAST
- 2 scrambled eggs and 2 grilled sausages

SNACK
- Celery sticks, almond butter and raisins

LUNCH
- 100g quinoa mixed with 2 boiled eggs, 1 chicken breast and broccoli

SNACK
- 1 can salmon

DINNER
- Homemade beef chilli with green vegetables and cauliflower rice (sauté a chopped onion for 10 minutes, then blend in a food processor with small florets of 1 cauliflower for 5-6 minutes)

SNACK
- Greek yoghurt with cinnamon and 10 walnuts

SUNDAY

BREAKFAST
- 2 poached eggs and smoked salmon

SNACK
- A handful of brazil nuts

LUNCH
- Diced lamb grilled on skewers with diced green and red peppers, diced onion and cherry tomatoes, with 1 baked sweet potato

SNACK
- Ham and ½ avocado

DINNER
- Beetroot, spinach and goat's cheese salad

SNACK
- Greek yoghurt with cinnamon and 10 walnuts

SHAKE IT!
Protein shakes have been included on Monday, Wednesday and Friday because it's an effective way to plan your gym workouts. If you train on other days, have shakes after those sessions instead.

WORKOUTS

As in the first two weeks, do this week's three workouts in order, taking at least one day off between each one to allow your muscles time to recover. Try to work out on the same days as in the previous weeks too, and don't forget your high-intensity cardio session (see p110).

WEEK THREE UPPER BODY

	EXERCISE	SETS	REPS	TEMPO	REST
1A	Bench press	3	12	2010	10sec
1B	Cable lateral raise	3	10	2110	10sec
1C	Cable crossover	3	12	2110	10sec
1D	Cable overhead biceps curl	3	12	2110	90sec
2A	Wide lat pull-down	3	12	2110	10sec
2B	Lat pull-down	3	10	2110	10sec
2C	Standing cable row	3	12	2110	10sec
2D	Cable face pull	3	12	2110	90sec

(WORKOUT 1)

•• Perform the first sets of 1A, 1B, 1C and 1D, taking 10 seconds' rest between each. Then rest for 90 seconds and repeat until all three sets are completed.

•• Perform the first sets of 2A, 2B, 2C and 2D, taking 10 seconds' rest between each. Then rest for 90 seconds and repeat until all three sets are completed.

WEEK THREE ▸ LOWER BODY

		EXERCISE	SETS	REPS	TEMPO	REST
WORKOUT 2	1A	Squat	3	12	3010	10sec
	1B	Front squat	3	10	3010	10sec
	1C	Leg extension	3	12	2010	10sec
	1D	Hamstring curl	3	12	2010	120sec
	2A	Dumbbell side lunge	3	12	1010	10sec
	2B	Squat jump	3	12	X	10sec
	2C	Lunge jump	3	12	X	10sec
	2D	Bunny hop	3	15	X	90sec

•• Perform the first sets of 1A, 1B, 1C and 1D, taking 10 seconds' rest between each. Then rest for 120 seconds and repeat until all three sets are completed.

•• Perform the first sets of 2A, 2B, 2C and 2D, taking 10 seconds' rest between each. Then rest for 90 seconds and repeat until all three sets are completed.

WEEK THREE ▸ TOTAL BODY

		EXERCISE	SETS	REPS	TEMPO	REST
WORKOUT 3	1A	Rack deadlift	3	12	2110	10sec
	1B	Triceps dip	3	10	3010	10sec
	1C	Neutral-grip chin-up	3	10	3010	10sec
	1D	Hanging leg raise	3	15	1111	120sec
	2A	Kettlebell goblet squat	3	15	X	10sec
	2B	Kettlebell clean and press	3	15	X	10sec
	2C	Kettlebell clean	3	15	X	10sec
	2D	Kettlebell swing	3	25	X	120sec

•• Perform the first sets of 1A, 1B, 1C and 1D, taking 10 seconds' rest between each. Then rest for 120 seconds and repeat until all three sets are completed.

•• Perform the first sets of 2A, 2B, 2C and 2D, taking 10 seconds' rest between each. Then rest for 120 seconds and repeat until all three sets are completed.

1A Bench press

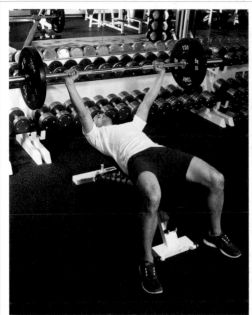
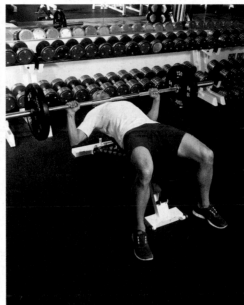

- Lie on a bench with your feet on the floor directly underneath your knees.
- Hold the bar with an overhand grip with your hands more than shoulder-width apart.
- Lower the bar towards your chest until your elbows are bent at 90° and the bar is almost touching the middle of your chest or is just above your nipples.
- Drive your feet hard into the floor and push the bar strongly back to the start.

1B Cable lateral raise

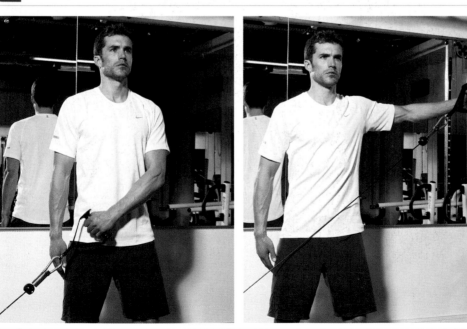

- Stand side-on to a cable machine, holding a D-handle attached to the low pulley in the hand farthest from the machine.
- Keeping a slight bend in your elbow, lift your arm up and away from the machine until it reaches shoulder height.
- Return slowly to the start.
- Complete all the required reps with that arm, then repeat with the other.

1C Cable crossover

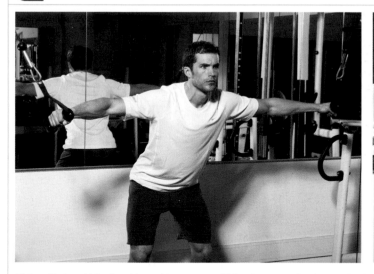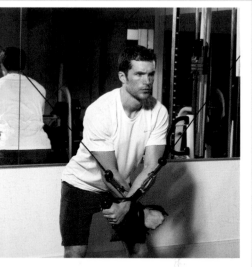

- Stand in the middle of a cable machine, holding a D-handle attachment in each hand with the cable set above shoulder height.
- Keeping a natural arch in your back, your core braced and your upper body still, bring your hands down in an arc to meet in front of your chest.
- At the bottom of the move squeeze your chest muscles and return slowly, and under full control of the weight, back to the start.

1D Cable overhead biceps curl

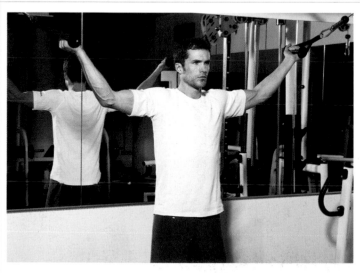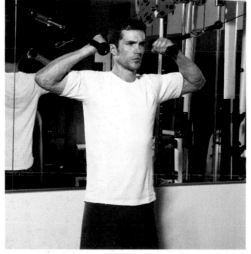

- Stand in the middle of a cable machine, holding a D-handle attached to the high pulley in each hand.
- Keeping your elbows steady, curl the handles towards your face.
- At the top of the move squeeze your biceps and return to the start.

2A Wide lat pull-down

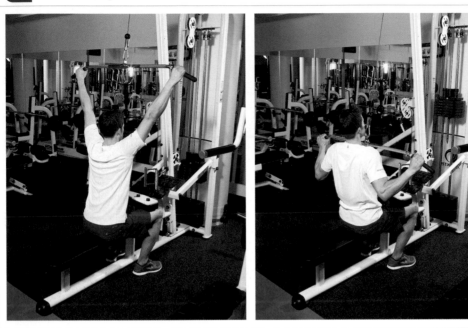

- Sit on the seat and take an overhand grip of the bar so your hands are double shoulder-width apart.
- Look forwards, retract your shoulder blades and keep your torso upright.
- Pull the bar down until it reaches your upper chest. Don't lean back to aid the movement.
- At the bottom of the move squeeze your lats and return to the start.

2B Lat pull-down

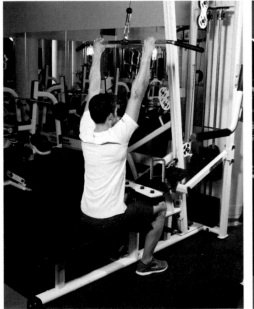
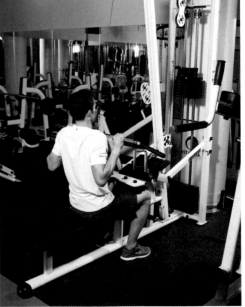

- Sit on the seat and take an overhand grip on the bar so your hands are shoulder-width apart.
- Look forwards, retract your shoulder blades and keep your torso upright.
- Pull the bar down until it reaches your upper chest. Don't lean back to aid the movement.
- At the bottom of the move squeeze your lats and return to the start.

2C Standing cable row

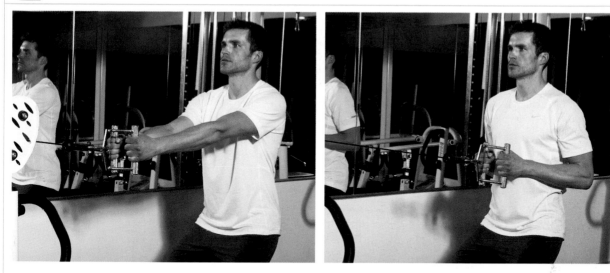

■ Stand facing a cable machine with your knees slightly bent, holding a double-D handle with a neutral grip attached to the middle pulley.

■ Ensure there's tension in the cable. Pull the handle into your sternum, keeping upper-body movement to a minimum.

■ At the top of the move squeeze your shoulder blades together and return slowly to the start.

2D Cable face pull

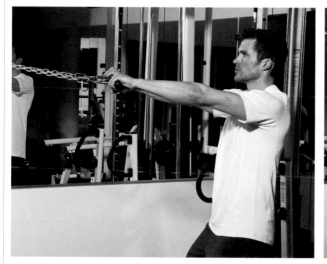

■ Stand facing a cable machine, holding a double-rope handle with an overhand grip attached to the high pulley. Your arms should be fully extended.

■ Pull the handles towards you, keeping your upper arms parallel to the floor, so the handles go either side of your face.

■ Return slowly to the start.

FAT-LOSS FINISHER
Kettlebell swing
p173

1A Squat

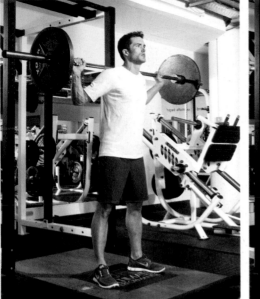
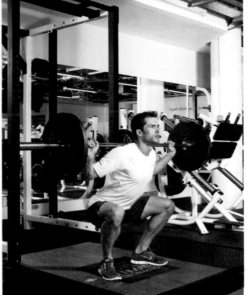

- Rest a barbell on the back of your shoulders – not your neck – holding it with an overhand grip slightly wider than your shoulders. Keep your elbows pointing to the floor.
- Your feet should be slightly more than shoulder-width apart with your toes pointing outwards slightly.
- Squat until your thighs are at least parallel to the floor, keeping your knees in line with your toes.
- Push back up through your heels to return to the start.

1B Front squat

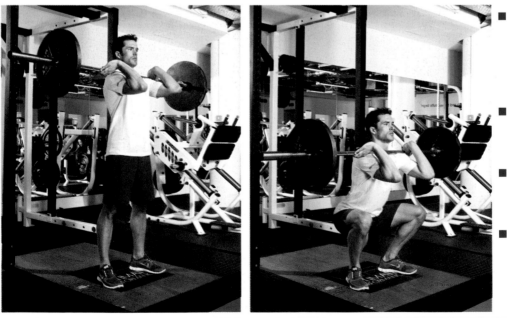

- Rest a barbell on the front of your shoulders, holding it with an overhand grip slightly wider than your shoulders. Keep your elbows pointing forwards.
- Your feet should be slightly more than shoulder-width apart with your toes pointing outwards slightly.
- Squat until your thighs are at least parallel to the floor, keeping your knees in line with your toes.
- Push back up through your heels to return to the start.

1C Leg extension

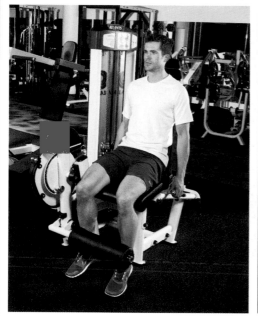

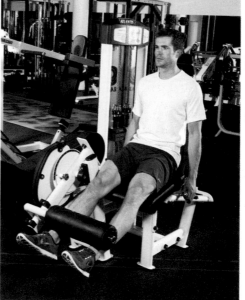

- Sit on the machine, following the instructions to position yourself correctly and safely.
- With the pad against the lower part of your shins, straighten your legs to raise it.
- Return slowly to the start.

1D Hamstring curl

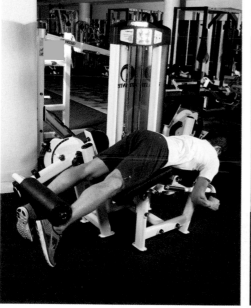
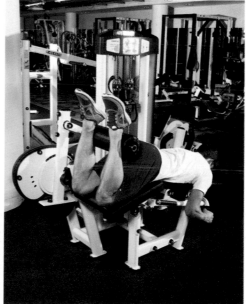

- Lie on your front on the machine, following the instructions to position yourself correctly and safely.
- With the pad against your lower calves, bend your knees and contract your hamstrings to raise it.
- Return slowly to the start.

2A Dumbbell side lunge

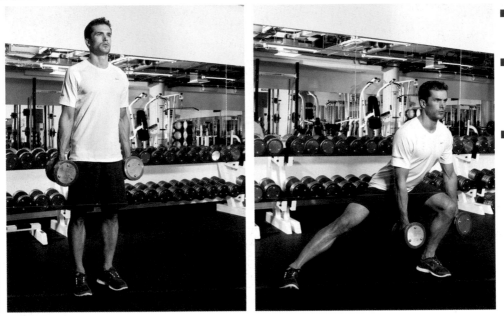

- Stand tall with your feet close together, holding a dumbbell in each hand by your sides.
- Keeping your core braced and your head looking forwards, take a big step to one side and lower your body towards the leading leg.
- Push back off the leg to return to the start and repeat the other side. That's one rep.

2B Squat jump

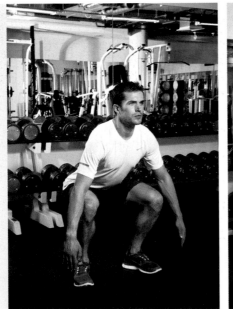
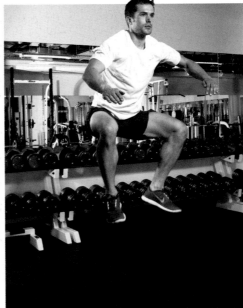

- Stand tall with your feet shoulder-width apart and your core braced.
- Squat until your thighs are at least parallel to the floor, keeping your knees in line with your toes.
- Push off the ground explosively so both feet leave the floor.
- As you land, descend straight into the next rep.

2C Lunge jump

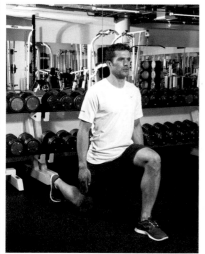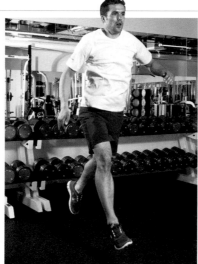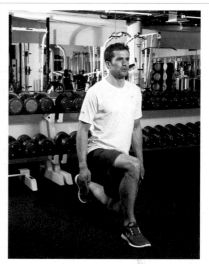

- Stand tall with your feet close together. Take a big step forwards with one leg and lunge until both knees are bent at 90°.
- Push back off your front foot explosively so both feet leave the ground. Swap feet mid-air, so you land with your other foot forwards.
- Descend straight into another lunge. Swap your legs with each rep.

2D Bunny hop

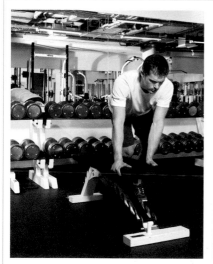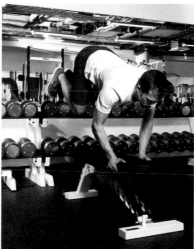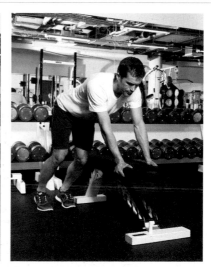

- Stand on one side of a bench with your feet together. Bend at the hips and grip either side of the bench.
- Push off the floor explosively to lift your legs up and over the bench.
- When you land, push back off and return to the start. That's one rep.

FAT-LOSS FINISHER
Sprint
p175

1A Rack deadlift

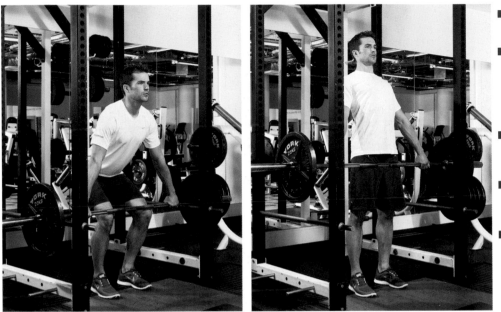

- Set the safety bars on a squat rack to mid-knee level.
- With the barbell resting on the bars, take a wide grip. Make sure your core is braced, your shoulders are retracted and over the bar, and your back is flat.
- Use your glutes to power the initial lift, pushing down through your heels.
- Keep the bar close to your body. As it passes your knees, push your hips forwards.
- Lower the weight so it just touches the bars before performing the next rep.

1B Triceps dip

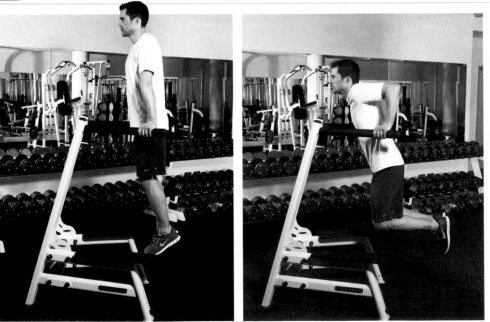

- Grip parallel bars, keeping your body upright.
- With your elbows pointing straight back, lower your body as far as you can comfortably go without stressing your shoulders.
- Keep your core braced and don't swing your legs for momentum.
- Press back up powerfully to return to the start, but don't lock out your elbows at the top of the move.

1C Neutral-grip chin-up

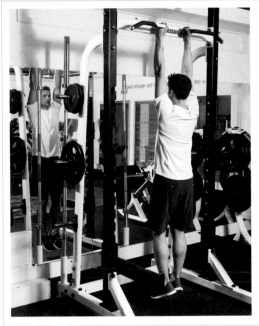

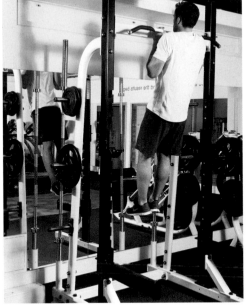

- Hold the bar so your hands are shoulder-width apart and your palms are facing each other.
- Start from a dead hang with your arms fully extended.
- Squeeze your lats together and pull yourself up.
- Once your chin is higher than your hands, lower yourself back to the start.

1D Hanging leg raise

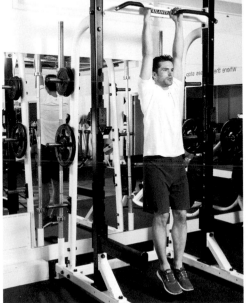

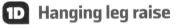

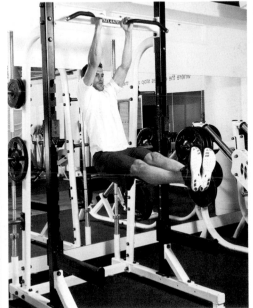

- Hang from a bar with your body straight.
- Keeping your legs straight, use your lower abs to raise them until they're parallel to the floor.

2A Kettlebell goblet squat

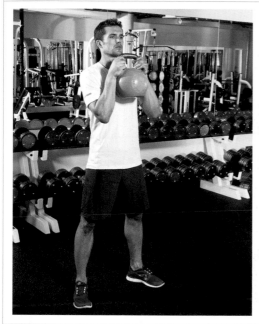
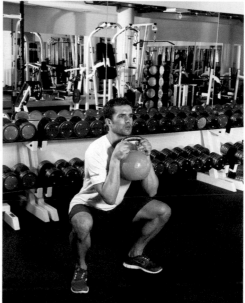

- Stand tall with your feet hip-width apart, holding a kettlebell in both hands in front of your upper chest.
- Keeping your core braced and a natural arch in your back, squat until your thighs are at least parallel to the floor. The deeper you can squat, the better.
- Push back through your heels to return to the start.

2B Kettlebell clean and press

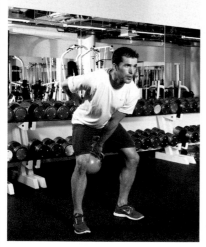
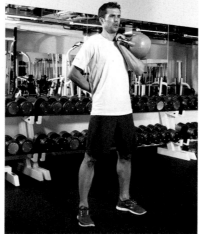
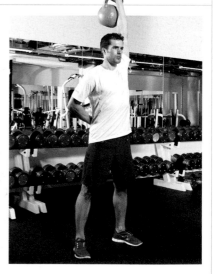

- Stand holding a kettlebell in one hand. Bend your knees slightly and swing the kettlebell back between your legs, then swing it upwards with a pop from your hips.

- Bend your elbow and let the handle slide into the base of your palm to rack the kettlebell on the front of your shoulder, keeping your elbow close to your body.

- Keeping your core braced, press the weight directly overhead. Reverse the move to return to the start. Complete half the required reps, then swap arms and repeat.

2C Kettlebell clean

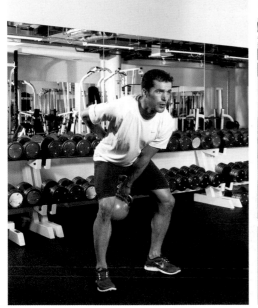
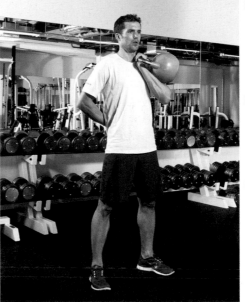

- Stand holding a kettlebell in one hand. Bend your knees slightly and swing the kettlebell back between your legs, then swing it upwards with a pop from your hips.

- Bend your elbow and let the handle slide into the base of your palm to rack the kettlebell on the front of your shoulder, keeping your elbow close to your body.

- Reverse the move to return to the start. Complete half the required reps, then swap arms and repeat.

2D Kettlebell swing

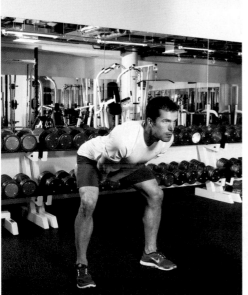
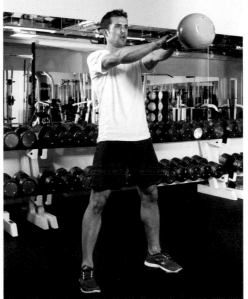

- Stand with your feet shoulder-width apart, holding a kettlebell in both hands.

- Keeping your back straight and your knees in line with your feet, bend your knees and swing the kettlebell between your legs.

- Brace your core, stand up and snap your hips forwards to propel the kettlebell up to shoulder height. The power comes from your hips, not your arms.

- Continue the swing in a fluid, controlled movement for the required number of reps.

FAT-LOSS FINISHER
Sled drag
p176

GET MOVING

Choose your activity to complete this week's training programme

The fourth and final session of week three is a 25-minute high-intensity cardio session. Whether you run, cycle or row is up to you. To complete the session, simply follow the charts below to make sure you work your muscles and cardiovascular system to burn the optimum amount of body fat.

RUN | BIKE | ROW

DURATION	INTENSITY	DURATION	INTENSITY	DURATION	INTENSITY
5min	2	5min	2	5min	2
5min	3	5min	3	5min	3
30sec	4	30sec	4	30sec	4
1min	3	1min	3	1min	3
30sec	4	30sec	4	30sec	4
1min	3	1min	3	1min	3
30sec	4	30sec	4	30sec	4
45sec	3	45sec	3	45sec	3
45sec	4	45sec	4	45sec	4
30sec	3	30sec	3	30sec	3
45sec	4	45sec	4	45sec	4
15sec	5	15sec	5	15sec	5
1min	2	1min	2	1min	2
45sec	4	45sec	4	45sec	4
15sec	5	15sec	5	15sec	5
30sec	3	30sec	3	30sec	3
45sec	4	45sec	4	45sec	4
15sec	5	15sec	5	15sec	5
3min	3	3min	3	3min	3
1min	2	1min	2	1min	2
1min	1	1min	1	1min	1

HOW HARD SHOULD YOU WORK?

Use this key to discover how much effort you should put in during every interval

1 Easy	2 Comfortable	3 Moderate	4 Intense	5 All-out

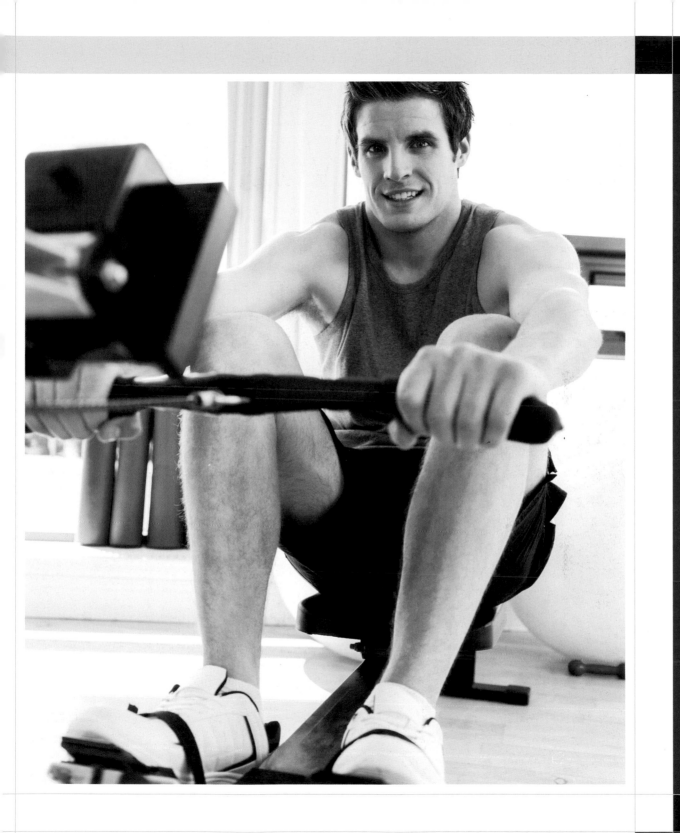

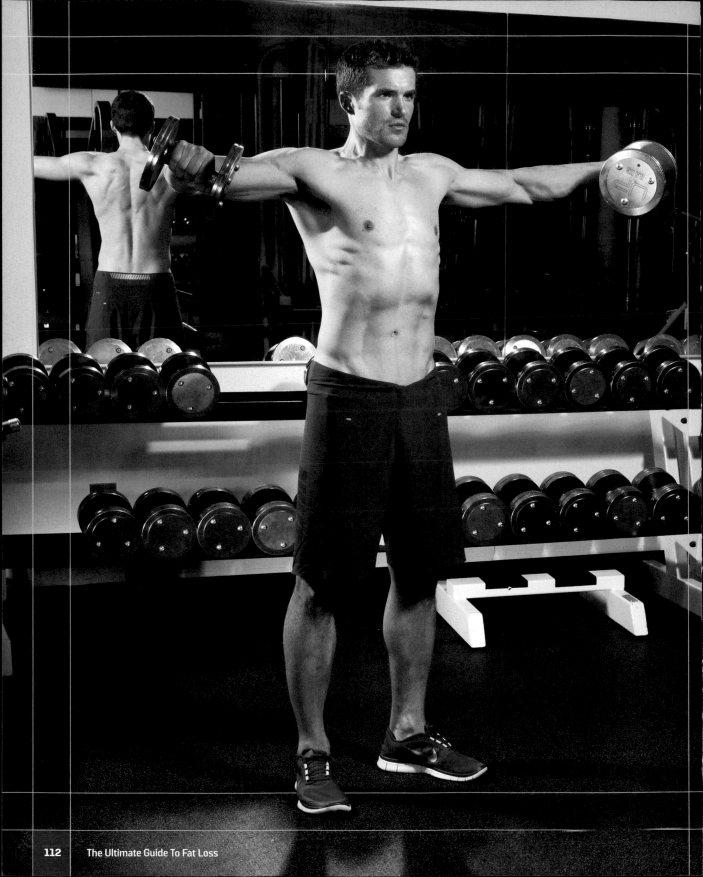

WEEK FOUR

Turn the page for the **fourth week** of your **six-week** nutrition and exercise plan

THIS WEEK'S MENU

MONDAY	TUESDAY	WEDNESDAY	THURSDAY
BREAKFAST ■ Spinach and goat's cheese omelette with a handful of almonds	**BREAKFAST** ■ Roast beef slices with wilted spinach and asparagus	**BREAKFAST** ■ 2 boiled eggs and 1 slice rye bread	**BREAKFAST** ■ 2 grilled venison sausages and 2 scrambled eggs
SNACK ■ Post-workout shake: blend 150ml almond milk, 1 scoop chocolate whey protein powder, ½ banana and 2tbsp Greek yoghurt	**SNACK** ■ Pineapple slices and cottage cheese	**SNACK** ■ Post-workout shake: blend 150ml almond milk, 1 scoop chocolate whey protein powder, ½ banana and 2tbsp Greek yoghurt	**SNACK** ■ Pineapple slices and cottage cheese
LUNCH ■ 150g couscous and 150g Greek salad with sundried tomatoes, cucumber, red onion, feta cheese, 15 olives, ½ chilli and 1 pepper	**LUNCH** ■ Grilled chicken breast with mixed salad and ½ avocado	**LUNCH** ■ 200g can tuna mixed with 2tsp chickpeas, lettuce, cucumber, spring onion, carrot, coriander, 30g (dry weight) cooked brown rice, olive oil and balsamic vinegar	**LUNCH** ■ ½ carton carrot and coriander soup with steamed green vegetables
SNACK ■ 1 carrot, 100g sliced green and red pepper	**SNACK** ■ 1 banana and a handful of almonds	**SNACK** ■ Apple and a handful of pumpkin seeds	**SNACK** ■ 1 banana and a handful of almonds
DINNER ■ Grilled chicken breast with chilli sauce and roasted vegetables	**DINNER** ■ 120g tuna steak, stir-fried broccoli, green beans and spinach	**DINNER** ■ 120g salmon, stir-fried broccoli, green beans, red pepper and spinach	**DINNER** ■ Large chicken salad with toasted walnuts
SNACK ■ 115g cottage cheese and 2 wholegrain rice cakes	**SNACK** ■ Greek yoghurt and blueberries	**SNACK** ■ 115g cottage cheese and 2 wholegrain rice cakes	**SNACK** ■ Greek yoghurt with cinnamon and 6 brazil nuts

Here's what you need to eat and when over the next seven days to blast away body fat

FRIDAY	SATURDAY	SUNDAY
BREAKFAST ▪ Roast chicken slices with mixed vegetables and a handful of nuts	**BREAKFAST** ▪ 2 scrambled eggs, ½ can cooked tomatoes, ½ can reduced salt and sugar beans, mushrooms and 2 rashers grilled bacon	**BREAKFAST** ▪ 2 scrambled eggs, ½ can cooked tomatoes, ½ can reduced salt and sugar beans, mushrooms and 2 rashers grilled bacon
SNACK ▪ Post-workout shake: blend 150ml almond milk, 1 scoop chocolate whey protein powder, ½ banana and 2tbsp Greek yoghurt	**SNACK** ▪ Pineapple slices and cottage cheese	**SNACK** ▪ A handful of almonds and raisins
LUNCH ▪ Ham and avocado salad	**LUNCH** ▪ Tuna salad with cherry tomatoes and beetroot	**LUNCH** ▪ ½ carton of carrot and coriander soup with steamed green vegetables
SNACK ▪ A handful of almonds, raisins and dark chocolate chips	**SNACK** ▪ 1 banana and a handful of almonds	**SNACK** ▪ Hummus with carrot sticks and 100g sliced green and red peppers
DINNER ▪ Beef fajitas: 100g fillet steak cut into strips with 1 red, 1 green pepper and 2 tortilla wraps	**DINNER** ▪ 200g salmon teriyaki with spinach and steamed courgette slices	**DINNER** ▪ Roast beef, sweet potato mash, carrots, spinach, broccoli and parsnips
SNACK ▪ 115g cottage cheese and 2 wholegrain rice cakes	**SNACK** ▪ Greek yoghurt with cinnamon and 6 brazil nuts	**SNACK** ▪ 115g cottage cheese on 2 wholegrain rice cakes

SHAKE IT!
Protein shakes have been included on Monday, Wednesday and Friday because it's an effective way to plan your gym workouts. If you train on other days, have shakes after those sessions instead.

WORKOUTS

Now you're over the halfway point, you should have established a rhythm to your week – doing the workouts in order and leaving at least a day's rest in between each one. Continue to follow this pattern and don't forget to include your high-intensity cardio session (see p130) at the end of the week.

WEEK FOUR ▶	UPPER BODY				
	EXERCISE	SETS	REPS	TEMPO	REST
1A	Bench press	4	10	2010	10sec
1B	Cable lateral raise	4	8	2110	10sec
1C	Cable crossover	4	10	2110	10sec
1D	Cable overhead biceps curl	4	10	2110	90sec
2A	Wide lat pull-down	4	10	2110	10sec
2B	Lat pull-down	4	8	2110	10sec
2C	Standing cable row	4	10	2110	10sec
2D	Cable face pull	4	10	2110	90sec

(WORKOUT 1)

•• Perform the first sets of 1A, 1B, 1C and 1D, taking 10 seconds' rest between each. Then rest for 90 seconds and repeat until all four sets are completed.

•• Perform the first sets of 2A, 2B, 2C and 2D, taking 10 seconds' rest between each. Then rest for 90 seconds and repeat until all four sets are completed.

WEEK FOUR   LOWER BODY

WORKOUT 2

	EXERCISE	SETS	REPS	TEMPO	REST
1A	Squat	4	10	3010	10sec
1B	Front squat	4	8	3010	10sec
1C	Leg extension	4	10	2010	10sec
1D	Hamstring curl	4	10	2010	120sec
2A	Dumbbell side lunge	4	10	1010	10sec
2B	Squat jump	4	10	X	10sec
2C	Lunge jump	4	10	X	10sec
2D	Bunny hop	4	12	X	90sec

•• Perform the first sets of 2A, 2B, 2C and 2D, taking 10 seconds' rest between each. Then rest for 120 seconds and repeat until all four sets are completed.

•• Perform the first sets of 2A, 2B, 2C and 2D, taking 10 seconds' rest between each. Then rest for 90 seconds and repeat until all four sets are completed.

WEEK FOUR   TOTAL BODY

WORKOUT 3

	EXERCISE	SETS	REPS	TEMPO	REST
1A	Rack deadlift	4	10	2110	10sec
1B	Triceps dip	4	8	3010	10sec
1C	Neutral-grip chin-up	4	8	3010	10sec
1D	Hanging leg raise	4	12	1111	120sec
2A	Kettlebell goblet squat	4	12	X	10sec
2B	Kettlebell clean and press	4	12	X	10sec
2C	Kettlebell clean	4	12	X	10sec
2D	Kettlebell swing	4	20	X	120sec

•• Perform the first sets of 1A, 1B, 1C and 1D, taking 10 seconds' rest between each. Then rest for 120 seconds and repeat until all four sets are completed.

•• Perform the first sets of 2A, 2B, 2C and 2D, taking 10 seconds' rest between each. Then rest for 120 seconds and repeat until all four sets are completed.

1A Bench press

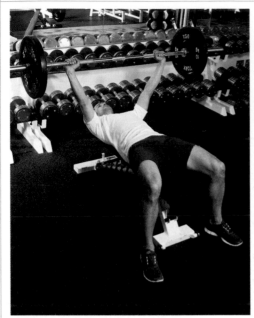 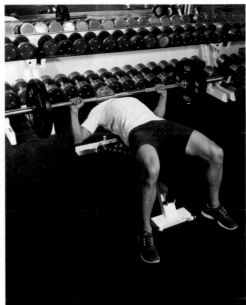

- Lie on a bench with your feet on the floor directly underneath your knees.
- Hold the bar with an overhand grip with your hands more than shoulder-width apart.
- Lower the bar towards your chest until your elbows are bent at 90° and the bar is almost touching the middle of your chest or is just above your nipples.
- Drive your feet hard into the floor and push the bar strongly back to the start.

1B Cable lateral raise

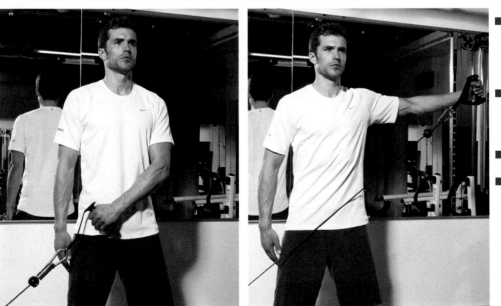

- Stand side-on to a cable machine, holding a D-handle attached to the low pulley in the hand farthest from the machine.
- Keeping a slight bend in your elbow, lift your arm up and away from the machine until it reaches shoulder height.
- Return slowly to the start.
- Complete all the required reps with that arm, then repeat with the other.

1C Cable crossover

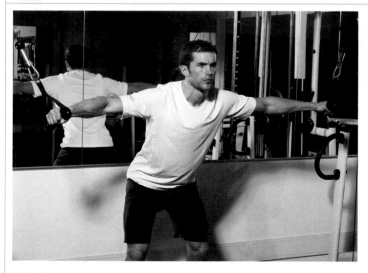
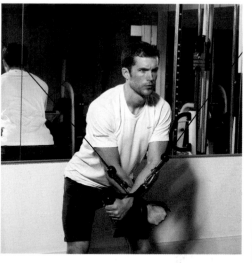

- Stand in the middle of a cable machine, holding a D-handle attachment in each hand with the cable set above shoulder height.
- Keeping a natural arch in your back, your core braced and your upper body still, bring your hands down in an arc to meet in front of your chest.
- At the bottom of the move squeeze your chest muscles and return slowly, and under full control of the weight, back to the start.

1D Cable overhead biceps curl

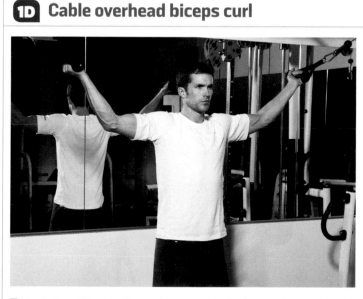
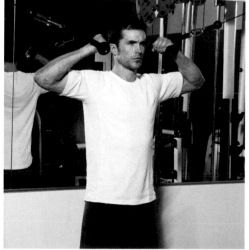

- Stand in the middle of a cable machine, holding a D-handle attached to the high pulley in each hand.
- Keeping your elbows steady, curl the handles towards your face.
- At the top of the move squeeze your biceps and return to the start.

2A Wide lat pull-down

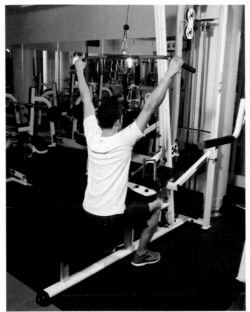 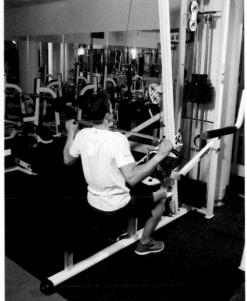

- Sit on the seat and take an overhand grip of the bar so your hands are double shoulder-width apart.
- Look forwards, retract your shoulder blades and keep your torso upright.
- Pull the bar down until it reaches your upper chest. Don't lean back to aid the movement.
- At the bottom of the move squeeze your lats and return to the start.

2B Lat pull-down

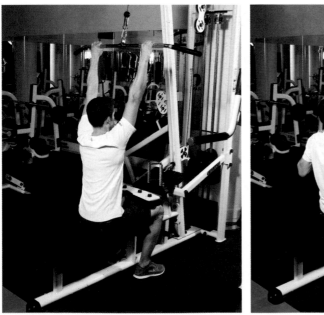 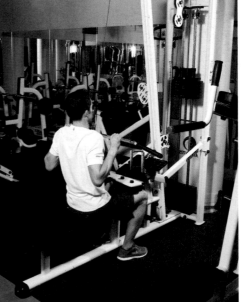

- Sit on the seat and take an overhand grip on the bar so your hands are shoulder-width apart.
- Look forwards, retract your shoulder blades and keep your torso upright.
- Pull the bar down until it reaches your upper chest. Don't lean back to aid the movement.
- At the bottom of the move squeeze your lats and return to the start.

2C   Standing cable row

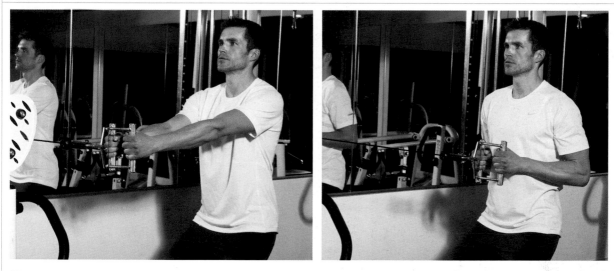

- Stand facing a cable machine with your knees slightly bent, holding a double-D handle with a neutral grip attached to the middle pulley.
- Ensure there's tension in the cable. Pull the handle into your sternum, keeping upper-body movement to a minimum.
- At the top of the move squeeze your shoulder blades together and return slowly to the start.

2D   Cable face pull

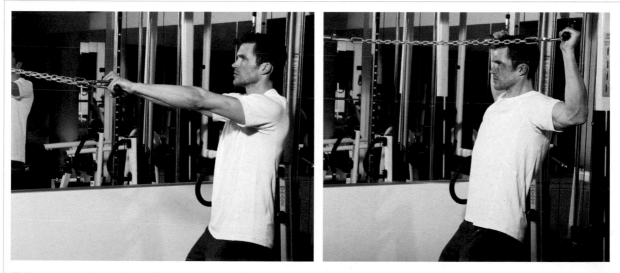

- Stand facing a cable machine, holding a double-rope handle with an overhand grip attached to the high pulley. Your arms should be fully extended.
- Pull the handles towards you, keeping your upper arms parallel to the floor, so the handles go either side of your face.
- Return slowly to the start.

FAT-LOSS FINISHER
Kettlebell swing
p173

1A Squat

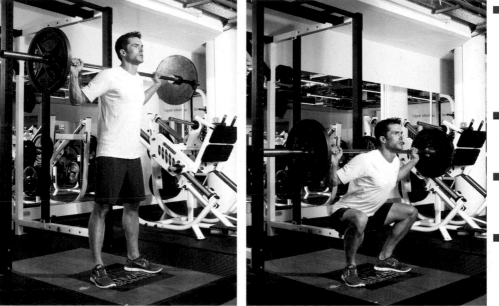

- Rest a barbell on the back of your shoulders – not your neck – holding it with an overhand grip slightly wider than your shoulders. Keep your elbows pointing to the floor.
- Your feet should be slightly more than shoulder-width apart with your toes pointing outwards slightly.
- Squat until your thighs are at least parallel to the floor, keeping your knees in line with your toes.
- Push back up through your heels to return to the start.

1B Front squat

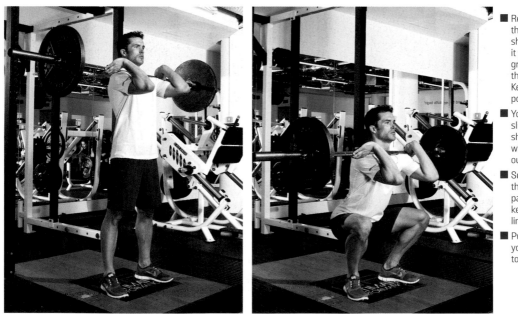

- Rest a barbell on the front of your shoulders, holding it with an overhand grip slightly wider than your shoulders. Keep your elbows pointing forwards.
- Your feet should be slightly more than shoulder-width apart with your toes pointing outwards slightly.
- Squat until your thighs are at least parallel to the floor, keeping your knees in line with your toes.
- Push back up through your heels to return to the start.

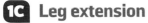 Leg extension

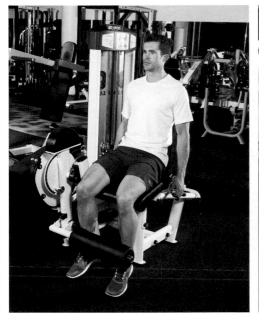 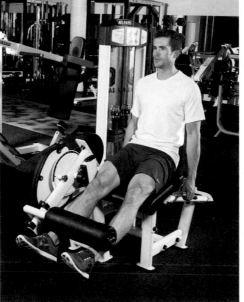

- Sit on the machine, following the instructions to position yourself correctly and safely.
- With the pad against the lower part of your shins, straighten your legs to raise it.
- Return slowly to the start.

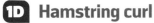 Hamstring curl

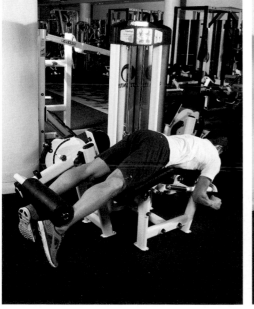 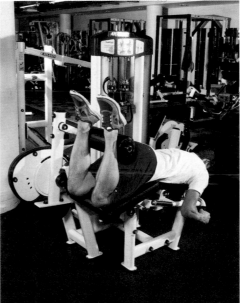

- Lie on your front on the machine, following the instructions to position yourself correctly and safely.
- With the pad against your lower calves, bend your knees and contract your hamstrings to raise it.
- Return slowly to the start.

2A Dumbbell side lunge

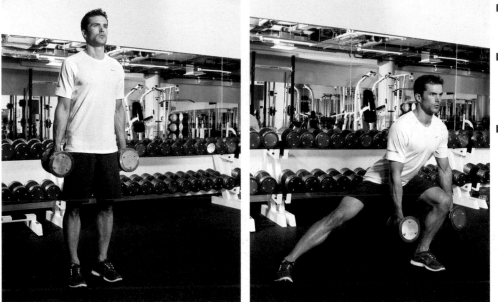

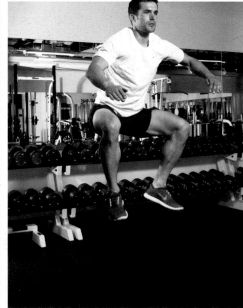

- Stand tall with your feet close together, holding a dumbbell in each hand by your sides.
- Keeping your core braced and your head looking forwards, take a big step to one side and lower your body towards the leading leg.
- Push back off the leg to return to the start and repeat the other side. That's one rep.

2B Squat jump

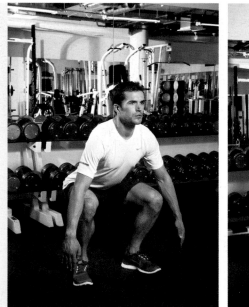

- Stand tall with your feet shoulder-width apart and your core braced.
- Squat until your thighs are at least parallel to the floor, keeping your knees in line with your toes.
- Push off the ground explosively so both feet leave the floor.
- As you land, descend straight into the next rep.

2C Lunge jump

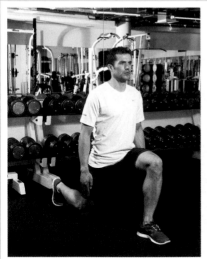 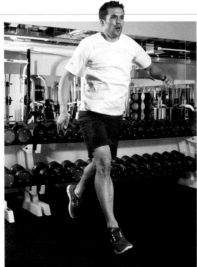 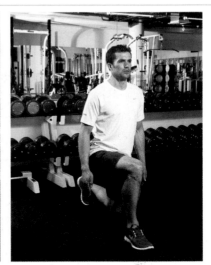

- Stand tall with your feet close together. Take a big step forwards with one leg and lunge until both knees are bent at 90°.

- Push back off your front foot explosively so both feet leave the ground. Swap feet mid-air, so you land with your other foot forwards.

- Descend straight into another lunge. Swap your legs with each rep.

2D Bunny hop

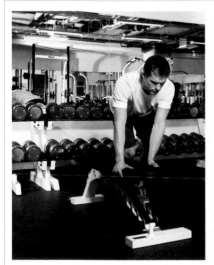 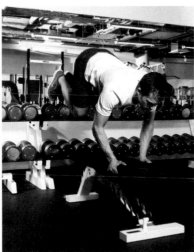 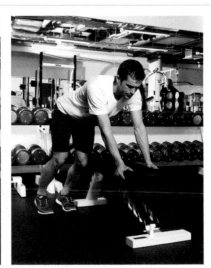

- Stand on one side of a bench with your feet together. Bend at the hips and grip either side of the bench.

- Push off the floor explosively to lift your legs up and over the bench.

- When you land, push back off and return to the start. That's one rep.

FAT-LOSS FINISHER Sprint p175

1A Rack deadlift

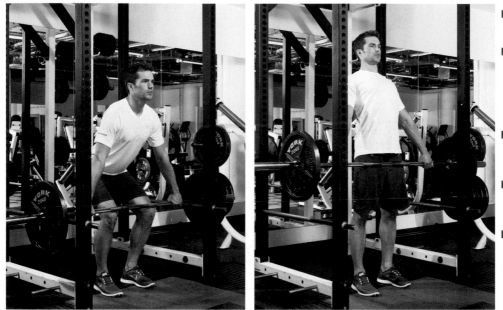

- Set the safety bars on a squat rack to mid-knee level.
- With the barbell resting on the bars, take a wide grip. Make sure your core is braced, your shoulders are retracted and over the bar, and your back is flat.
- Use your glutes to power the initial lift, pushing down through your heels.
- Keep the bar close to your body. As it passes your knees, push your hips forwards.
- Lower the weight so it just touches the bars before performing the next rep.

1B Triceps dip

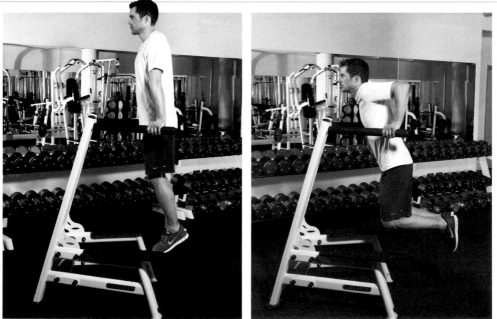

- Grip parallel bars, keeping your body upright.
- With your elbows pointing straight back, lower your body as far as you can comfortably go without stressing your shoulders.
- Keep your core braced and don't swing your legs for momentum.
- Press back up powerfully to return to the start, but don't lock out your elbows at the top of the move.

1C Neutral-grip chin-up

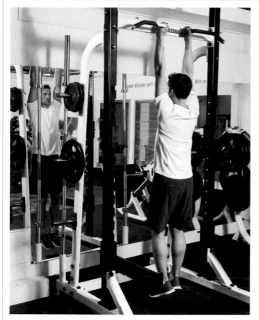
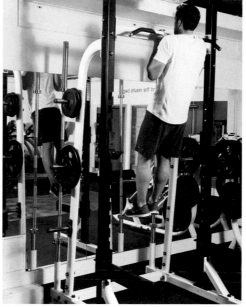

- Hold the bar so your hands are shoulder-width apart and your palms are facing each other.
- Start from a dead hang with your arms fully extended.
- Squeeze your lats together and pull yourself up.
- Once your chin is higher than your hands, lower yourself back to the start.

1D Hanging leg raise

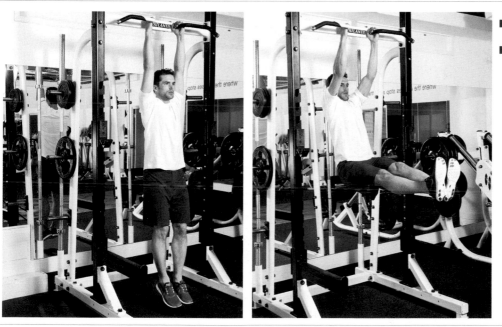
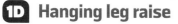

- Hang from a bar with your body straight.
- Keeping your legs straight, use your lower abs to raise them until they're parallel to the floor.

2A Kettlebell goblet squat

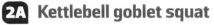

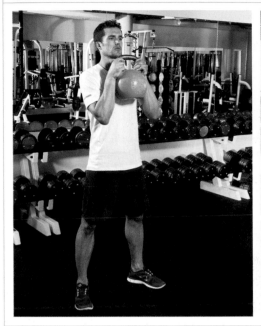

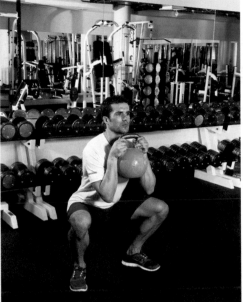

- Stand tall with your feet hip–width apart, holding a kettlebell in both hands in front of your upper chest.
- Keeping your core braced and a natural arch in your back, squat until your thighs are at least parallel to the floor. The deeper you can squat, the better.
- Push back through your heels to return to the start.

2B Kettlebell clean and press

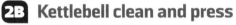

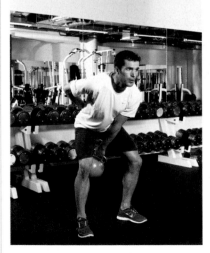

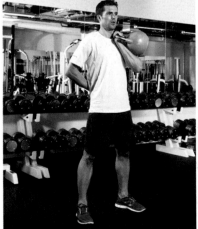

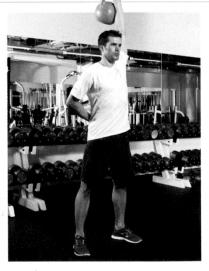

- Stand holding a kettlebell in one hand. Bend your knees slightly and swing the kettlebell back between your legs, then swing it upwards with a pop from your hips.

- Bend your elbow and let the handle slide into the base of your palm to rack the kettlebell on the front of your shoulder, keeping your elbow close to your body.

- Keeping your core braced, press the weight directly overhead. Reverse the move to return to the start. Complete half the required reps, then swap arms and repeat.

2C Kettlebell clean

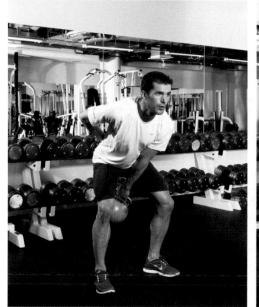
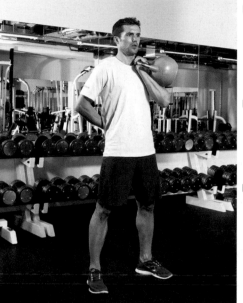

- Stand holding a kettlebell in one hand. Bend your knees slightly and swing the kettlebell back between your legs, then swing it upwards with a pop from your hips.

- Bend your elbow and let the handle slide into the base of your palm to rack the kettlebell on the front of your shoulder, keeping your elbow close to your body.

- Reverse the move to return to the start. Complete half the required reps, then swap arms and repeat.

2D Kettlebell swing

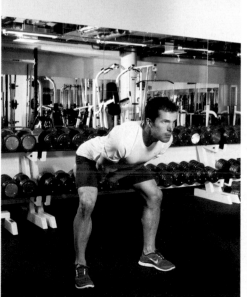
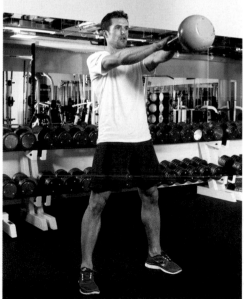

- Stand with your feet shoulder-width apart, holding a kettlebell in both hands.

- Keeping your back straight and your knees in line with your feet, bend your knees and swing the kettlebell between your legs.

- Brace your core, stand up and snap your hips forwards to propel the kettlebell up to shoulder height. The power comes from your hips, not your arms.

- Continue the swing in a fluid, controlled movement for the required number of reps.

FAT-LOSS FINISHER
Sled drag
p176

GET MOVING

Choose your activity to complete this week's training programme

The fourth and final session of week four is a 25-minute high-intensity cardio session. Whether you run, cycle or row is up to you. To complete the session, simply follow the charts below to make sure you work your muscles and cardiovascular system to burn the optimum amount of body fat.

🏃 RUN		🚴 BIKE		🚣 ROW	
DURATION	INTENSITY	DURATION	INTENSITY	DURATION	INTENSITY
5min	2	5min	2	5min	2
5min	3	5min	3	5min	3
30sec	4	30sec	4	30sec	4
30sec	3	30sec	3	30sec	3
30sec	4	30sec	4	30sec	4
30sec	3	30sec	3	30sec	3
1min	4	1min	4	1min	4
30sec	3	30sec	3	30sec	3
1min	4	1min	4	1min	4
30sec	3	30sec	3	30sec	3
1min	4	1min	4	1min	4
20sec	5	20sec	5	20sec	5
30sec	2	30sec	2	30sec	2
1min	4	1min	4	1min	4
20sec	5	20sec	5	20sec	5
30sec	2	30sec	2	30sec	2
1min	4	1min	4	1min	4
20sec	5	20sec	5	20sec	5
2min	3	2min	3	2min	3
2min	2	2min	2	2min	2
1min	1	1min	1	1min	1

HOW HARD SHOULD YOU WORK?

Use this key to discover how much effort you should put in during every interval

1 Easy	2 Comfortable	3 Moderate	4 Intense	5 All-out

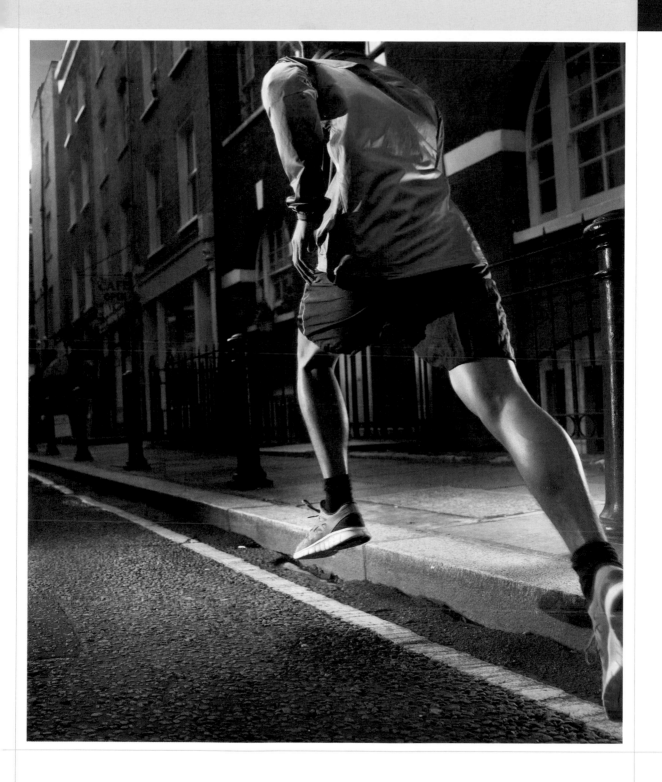

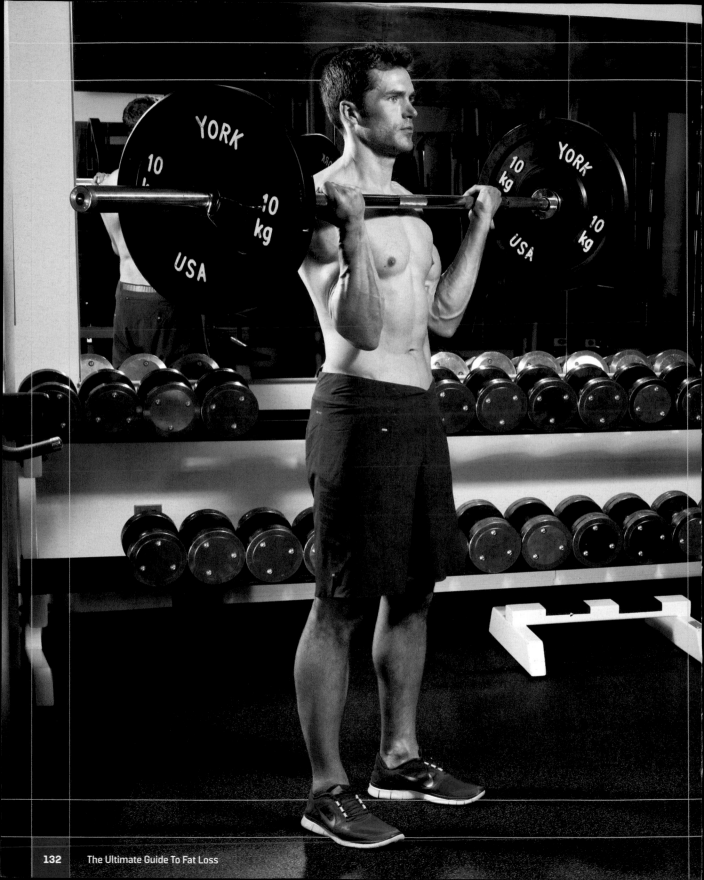

WEEK FIVE

Turn the page for the **fifth week** of your **six-week** nutrition and exercise plan

THIS WEEK'S MENU

MONDAY	TUESDAY	WEDNESDAY	THURSDAY
BREAKFAST ■ 2 grilled venison sausages and 2 scrambled eggs	**BREAKFAST** ■ Smoothie: blend 150ml coconut water, ½ frozen banana, a handful of spinach, 1tsp spirulina, 2tbsp coconut cream concentrate, 1tbsp ground flax meal and ice	**BREAKFAST** ■ Smoked haddock fillet, 2 poached eggs and asparagus	**BREAKFAST** ■ 3-egg omelette with mixed peppers and mushrooms
SNACK ■ Post-workout shake: blend 150ml coconut water, 1 scoop whey protein powder, 1 frozen banana, 1tbsp almond butter, 1tbsp ground flax seeds and ice	**SNACK** ■ Salsa with carrot and celery sticks	**SNACK** ■ Post-workout shake: blend 150ml coconut water, 1 scoop whey protein powder, 1 frozen banana, 1tbsp almond butter, 1tbsp ground flax seeds and ice	**SNACK** ■ 3 slices beef
LUNCH ■ Lamb burger, couscous and baby spinach salad	**LUNCH** ■ ½ carton broccoli and stilton soup with steamed green vegetables	**LUNCH** ■ Salmon fillet with asparagus, peas and a handful of spinach, drizzled with 2tbsp extra virgin olive oil and lemon juice	**LUNCH** ■ Tuna salad
SNACK ■ 2 plums and 12 almonds	**SNACK** ■ A handful of raisin and cashew nut mix	**SNACK** ■ 2 boiled eggs	**SNACK** ■ 1 apple and a handful of almonds
DINNER ■ Sweet and sour chicken with broccoli and cauliflower rice (sauté 1 chopped onion for 10 minutes, then blend in a food processor with small florets of 1 cauliflower for 5-6 minutes)	**DINNER** ■ Bolognese with courgette spaghetti	**DINNER** ■ Chicken breast with red pepper, cherry tomatoes, spinach, green beans, black olives and olive oil	**DINNER** ■ 120g salmon with stir-fried broccoli, green beans, red peppers and spinach, sesame seeds and olive oil
SNACK ■ Greek yoghurt with cinnamon	**SNACK** ■ Natural yoghurt with 1tsp honey and blackberries	**SNACK** ■ Greek yoghurt with cinnamon	**SNACK** ■ Natural yoghurt with 1tsp honey and blackberries

Here's what you need to eat and when over the next seven days to blast away body fat

FRIDAY	SATURDAY	SUNDAY
BREAKFAST ■ 2 rashers grilled bacon, 2 grilled tomatoes and 6 brazil nuts	**BREAKFAST** ■ Small steak, 2 poached eggs and asparagus	**BREAKFAST** ■ Roasted vegetable and goat's cheese omelette with a side salad
SNACK ■ Post-workout shake: blend 150ml coconut water, 1 scoop whey protein powder, 1 frozen banana, 1tbsp almond butter, 1tbsp ground flax seeds and ice	**SNACK** ■ ½ avocado and 2 slices ham	**SNACK** ■ Salsa with carrot and celery sticks
LUNCH ■ Lemon garlic chicken with steamed broccoli, avocado and pine nuts, drizzled with olive oil and lemon juice	**LUNCH** ■ Warm beetroot, goat's cheese and walnut salad	**LUNCH** ■ 1 grilled pork fillet and Greek salad
SNACK ■ 2 boiled eggs	**SNACK** ■ 1 banana and a handful of almonds	**SNACK** ■ 2 boiled eggs
DINNER ■ Red lentil and vegetable curry with 40g brown rice; 1 small glass red wine	**DINNER** ■ Baked salmon with roasted vegetables	**DINNER** ■ 2 grilled chicken breasts with grilled mixed vegetables
SNACK ■ Greek yoghurt with cinnamon	**SNACK** ■ Natural yoghurt with 1tsp honey and blackberries	**SNACK** ■ Natural yoghurt with 1tsp honey and blueberries

SHAKE IT!
Protein shakes have been included on Monday, Wednesday and Friday because it's an effective way to plan your gym workouts. If you train on other days, have shakes after those sessions instead.

WORKOUTS

Do the three workouts for week five in order, as in previous weeks, not forgetting to schedule a rest day between each session. Once you've completed all three workouts, remember to complete the high-intensity cardio routine (see p150).

WEEK FIVE UPPER BODY

	EXERCISE	SETS	REPS	TEMPO	REST
1A	Incline bench press	3	12	3010	10sec
1B	Shoulder press	3	10	3010	10sec
1C	Front raise	3	12	1010	10sec
1D	Lateral raise	3	12	1010	120sec
2A	Reverse-grip bent-over row	3	12	3010	10sec
2B	Chin-up	3	10	3010	10sec
2C	Cable reverse flye	3	12	2010	10sec
2D	Cable straight-arm pull-down	3	12	2010	90sec

WORKOUT 1

●● Perform the first sets of 1A, 1B, 1C and 1D, taking 10 seconds' rest between each. Then rest for 120 seconds and repeat until all three sets are completed.

●● Perform the first sets of 2A, 2B, 2C and 2D, taking 10 seconds' rest between each. Rest for 90 seconds and repeat until all three sets are completed.

WEEK FIVE — LOWER BODY

		EXERCISE	SETS	REPS	TEMPO	REST
WORKOUT 2	1A	Squat	3	12	2010	10sec
	1B	Lunge	3	12	2010	10sec
	1C	Calf raise	3	15	2110	10sec
	1D	Box jump	3	12	X	120sec
	2A	Hamstring curl	3	12	3010	10sec
	2B	Leg press	3	15	2010	0sec
	2C	Wide leg press	3	16	2010	0sec
	2D	Narrow leg press	3	15	2010	120sec

•• Perform the first sets of 1A, 1B, 1C and 1D, taking 10 seconds' rest between each. Then rest for 120 seconds and repeat until all three sets are completed.

•• Perform the first set of 2A, rest for 10 seconds, then do the first sets of 2B, 2C and 2D without taking any rest between each. Then rest for 120 seconds and repeat until all four sets are completed.

WEEK FIVE — TOTAL BODY

		EXERCISE	SETS	REPS	TEMPO	REST
WORKOUT 3	1A	Clean	3	12	X	10sec
	1B	Push press	3	10	3010	10sec
	1C	Romanian deadlift	3	12	2010	10sec
	1D	Barbell shrug	3	12	1110	90sec
	2A	Pull-up	3	8	3010	0sec
	2B	Hanging leg raise	3	15	1110	0sec
	2C	Hanging knee raise	3	15	1110	10sec
	2D	Barbell rollout	3	10	3110	90sec

•• Perform the first sets of 1A, 1B, 1C and 1D, taking 10 seconds' rest between each. Then rest for 120 seconds and repeat until all three sets are completed.

•• Perform the first sets of 2A, 2B and 2C without taking any rest between each. Rest for 10 seconds, then do the first set of 2D. Rest for 90 seconds and repeat until all three sets are completed.

1A Incline bench press

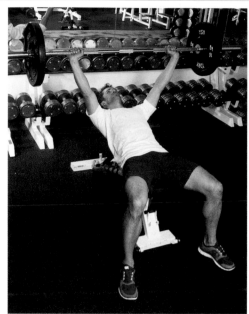
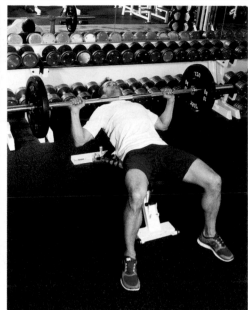

- Lie on a bench set at a 45° angle with your feet on the floor directly underneath your knees.
- Hold the bar with an overhand grip with your hands more than shoulder-width apart.
- Lower the bar towards your chest until your elbows are bent at 90° and the bar is almost touching the middle of your chest or is just above your nipples.
- Drive your feet hard into the floor and push the bar strongly back to the start.

1B Shoulder press

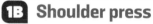
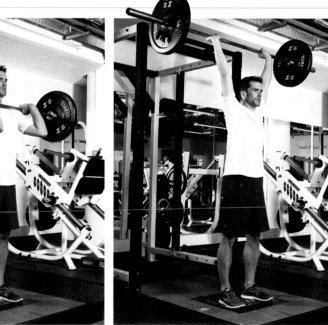

- Stand with your feet shoulder-width apart. Position a bar on your upper chest, gripping it with your hands slightly more than shoulder-width apart.
- Keep your chest upright and your core braced.
- Press the bar directly overhead until your arms are fully extended. Don't tilt your hips forwards.
- Lower the bar to return to the start.

1C Front raise

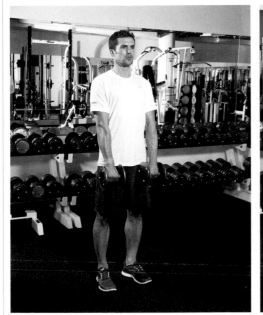 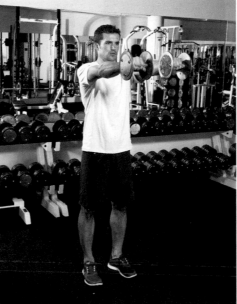

- Stand tall with your core braced and your feet shoulder-width apart, holding a light dumbbell in each hand in front of your thighs.
- Lift the weights in front of you, using your muscles and not momentum.
- Stop when the weights reach shoulder height. Lower to return to the start.

1D Lateral raise

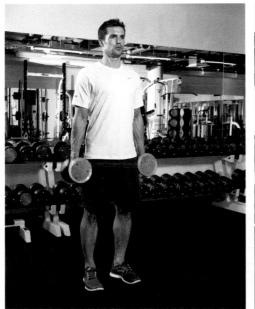 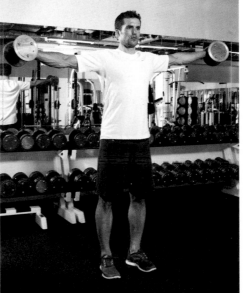

- Stand tall with your core braced and your feet shoulder-width apart, holding a light dumbbell in each hand by your sides with your palms facing your body.
- Leading with your elbows, lift the weights out to the sides, using your muscles and not momentum.
- Stop when the weights reach shoulder height. Lower to return to the start.

2A Reverse-grip bent-over row

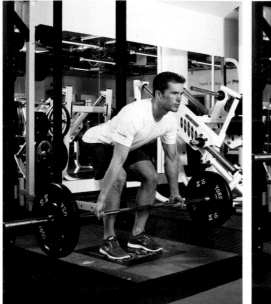
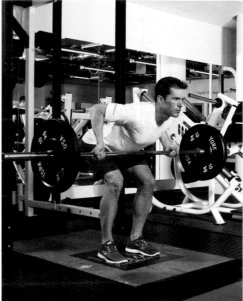

- Start with your core braced, your back straight and your shoulder blades retracted, gripping a bar with an underhand grip.
- Bend your knees slightly and lean forwards from the hips.
- Pull the bar up to your lower sternum, retracting your shoulder blades to allow the bar to come up to the chest, then lower again.

2B Chin-up

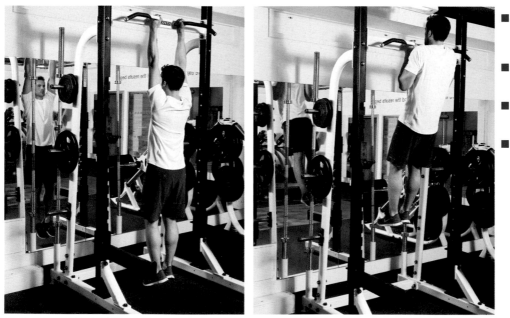

- Grab the bar with an underhand grip so your hands are shoulder-width apart.
- Start from a dead hang with your arms fully extended.
- Squeeze your lats together to pull yourself up.
- Once your chin is higher than your hands, lower yourself back to the start.

2C Cable reverse flye

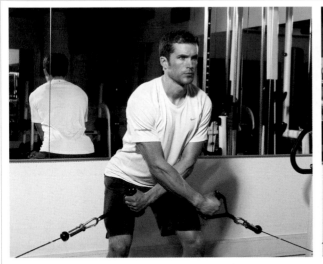

- Stand in the middle of a cable machine with your arms crossed, holding a D-handle attachment attached to the low pulley in each hand.
- Keeping your core braced and a slight bend in your elbows, lift both arms to shoulder height.
- Return to the start, maintaining control of the weight throughout.

2D Cable straight-arm pull-down

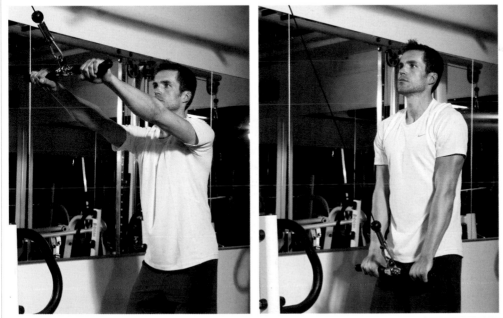

- Stand tall, holding a straight-bar handle attached to the high pulley of a cable machine.
- Keeping your arms straight, pull the bar down in an arc to your thighs.
- At the bottom of the move squeeze your lats and triceps and return to the start.

FAT-LOSS FINISHER
Burpee
p172

1A Squat

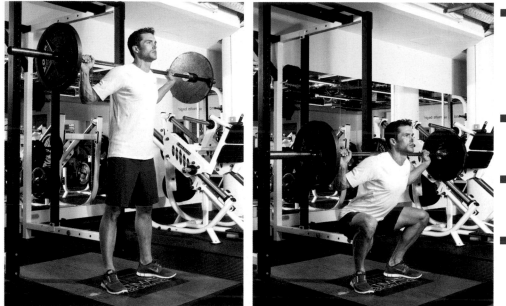

- Rest a barbell on the back of your shoulders – not your neck – holding it with an overhand grip slightly wider than your shoulders. Keep your elbows pointing to the floor.
- Your feet should be slightly more than shoulder width apart with your toes pointing outwards slightly.
- Squat until your thighs are at least parallel to the floor, keeping your knees in line with your toes.
- Push back up through your heels to return to the start.

1B Lunge

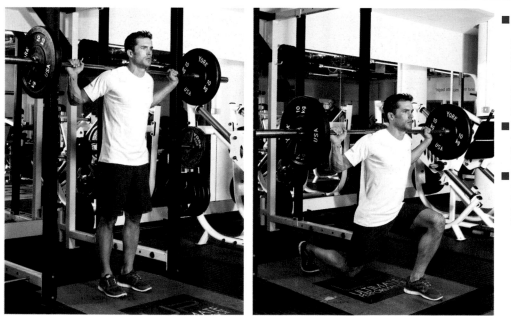

- Stand tall, resting a barbell on the back of your shoulders, not your neck. Point your elbows behind you to retract your shoulder blades, and keep your back upright and core braced throughout.
- Take a big step forwards with one leg and lunge until both knees are bent at 90°.
- Push back off your front foot to return to the start, then repeat with the other leg. That's one rep.

1C Calf raise

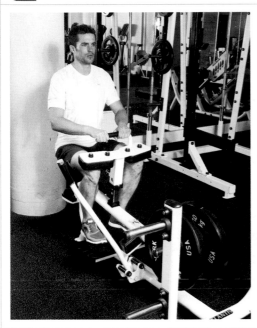 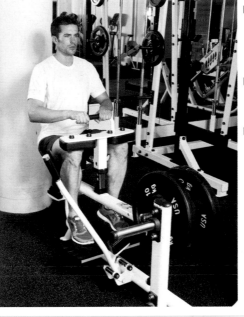

- Sit on the machine having adjusted the weight plates or stack, depending on the equipment, with your toes on the platform.
- Release the safety catch and go up on your tiptoes, keeping your body stable.
- Return to the start, making sure your heels go below the platform to achieve the full range of motion.

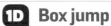 1D Box jump

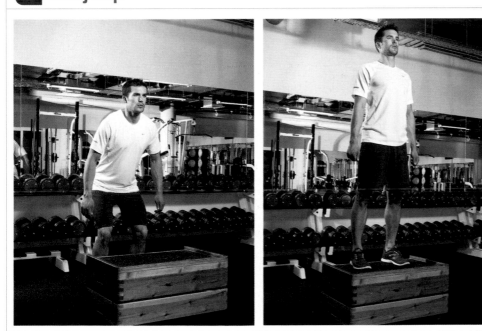

- Stand in front of a box or raised platform.
- Explosively jump on to the box, landing with both feet.
- Step back down to return to the start.

2A Hamstring curl

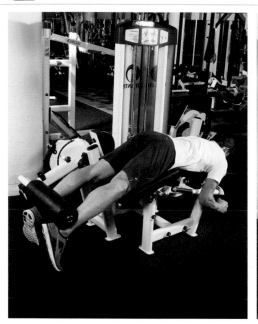 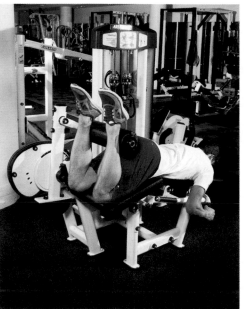

- Lie on your front on the machine, following the instructions to position yourself correctly and safely.
- With the pad against your lower calves, bend your knees and contract your hamstrings to raise it.
- Return to the start.

2B Leg press

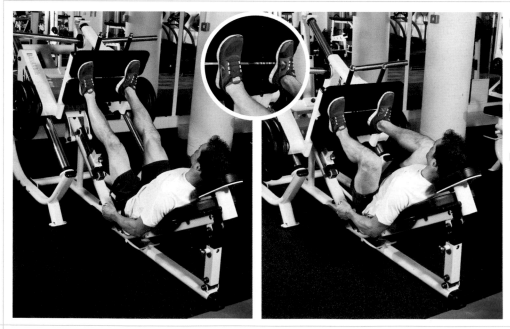

- Sit on the machine, following its instructions to position yourself correctly and safely, with your feet hip-width apart (see inset).
- Release the lock, bend your knees and slowly lower the platform towards you.
- Push through your heels to straighten your legs and return to the start.

2C Wide leg press

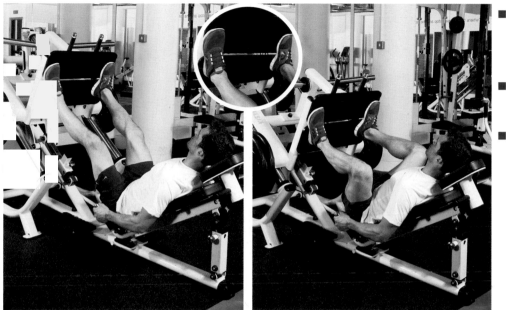

- Sit on the machine, following its instructions to position yourself correctly and safely, with your feet shoulder-width apart (see inset).
- Release the lock, bend your knees and slowly lower the platform towards you.
- Push through your heels to straighten your legs and return to the start.

2D Narrow leg press

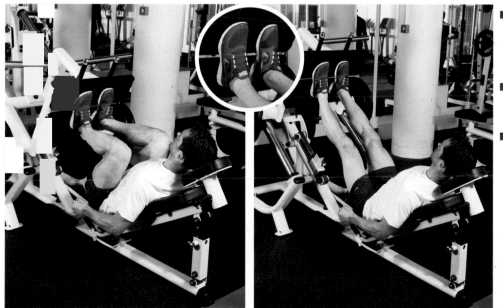

- Sit on the machine, following its instructions to position yourself correctly and safely, with your feet close together (see inset).
- Release the lock, bend your knees and slowly lower the platform towards you.
- Push through your heels to straighten your legs and return to the start.

FAT-LOSS FINISHER
Walking dumbbell lunge
p177

1A Clean

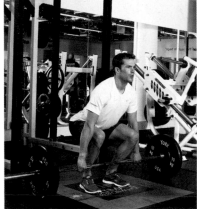 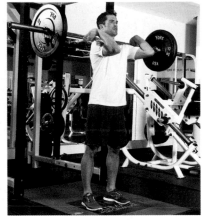

- Stand with your feet shoulder-width apart so your shins are touching the bar. Squat and take hold of the bar with an overhand grip.
- Keeping your core braced, your chest up and with a natural arch in your back, drive through your heels to lift the bar off the floor.

- As the bar reaches your hips, rise on to your tiptoes, shrug your shoulders and pull the bar up higher, leading with your elbows.
- As the bar travels towards your shoulders, squat under the bar and rotate your arms so your elbows face forwards

and you catch the bar on your fingers and the front of your shoulders.
- Reverse the move to return to the start.

1B Push press

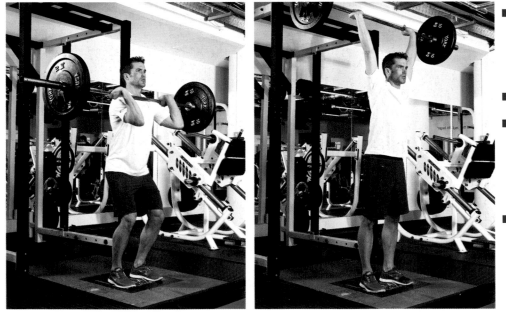

- Stand with your feet shoulder-width apart. Position a bar on your upper chest, holding it so your hands are slightly more than shoulder-width apart.
- Keep your chest upright and your core braced.
- Bend at the knees to go into a quarter-squat, then stand up and press the bar directly overhead until your arms are fully extended. Don't tilt your hips forwards.
- Lower the bar to return to the start.

1C Romanian deadlift

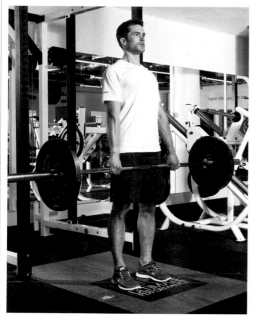 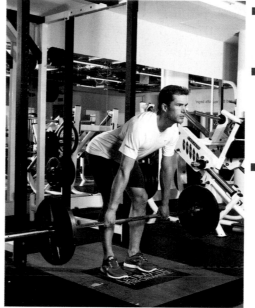

- Stand tall with your feet shoulder–width apart holding a barbell with an overhand grip just outside your thighs.

- Keeping a slight bend in your knees, lean forwards from your hips, not the waist, and lower the bar down the front of your shins until you feel a good stretch in your hamstrings.

- Reverse the move back to the start, pushing your hips forwards as you do so.

1D Barbell shrug

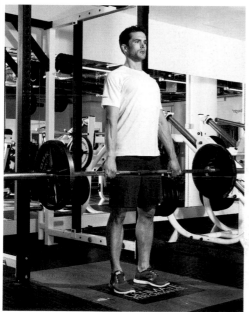 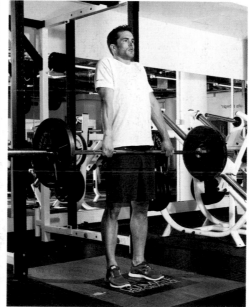

- Stand tall with your feet shoulder–width apart holding a barbell with an overhand grip just outside your thighs.

- Keeping your core braced and arms straight, shrug your shoulders towards your ears.

- Lower the weight back to the start.

2A Pull-up

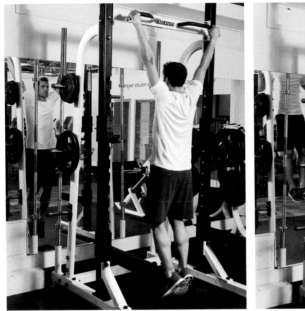
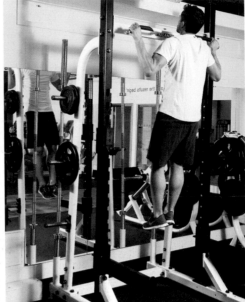

- Grab the bar with an overhand grip so your hands are more than shoulder-width apart.
- Start from a dead hang with your arms fully extended.
- Squeeze your lats together to pull yourself up.
- Once your chin is higher than your hands, lower yourself back to the start.

2B Hanging leg raise

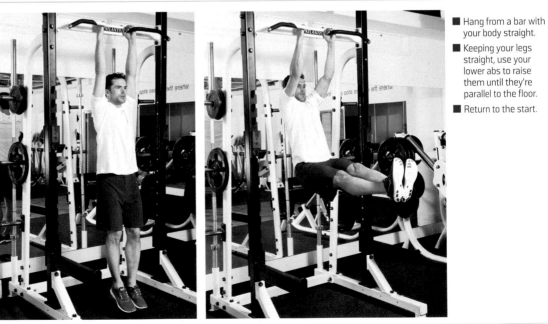

- Hang from a bar with your body straight.
- Keeping your legs straight, use your lower abs to raise them until they're parallel to the floor.
- Return to the start.

2C Hanging knee raise

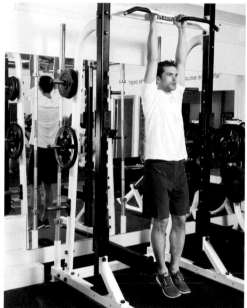
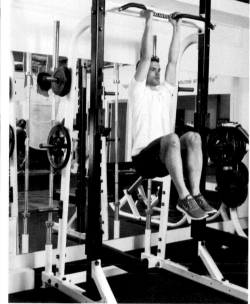

- Hang from a bar with your body straight.
- Bend your knees and use your lower abs to raise your legs until your thighs are parallel to the floor.
- Return to the start.

2D Barbell rollout

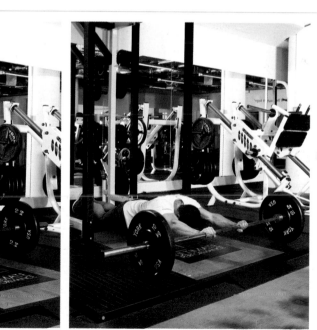

- Start on your knees with your arms extended and your hands holding a barbell with a shoulder-width grip.
- Roll the barbell away from your body, keeping your core braced.
- Once your torso is parallel to the floor, contract your abs and pull the bar back towards your body to return to the start.

FAT-LOSS FINISHER
Kettlebell swing
p173

GET MOVING

Choose your activity to complete this week's training programme

The fourth and final session of week five is a 25-minute high-intensity cardio session. Whether you run, cycle or row is up to you. To complete the session, simply follow the charts below to make sure you work your muscles and cardiovascular system to burn the optimum amount of body fat.

RUN		BIKE		ROW	
DURATION	INTENSITY	DURATION	INTENSITY	DURATION	INTENSITY
5min	2	5min	2	5min	2
5min	3	5min	3	5min	3
30sec	4	30sec	4	30sec	4
30sec	3	30sec	3	30sec	3
30sec	4	30sec	4	30sec	4
30sec	3	30sec	3	30sec	3
1min	4	1min	4	1min	4
30sec	3	30sec	3	30sec	3
1min	4	1min	4	1min	4
30sec	3	30sec	3	30sec	3
1min	4	1min	4	1min	4
20sec	5	20sec	5	20sec	5
30sec	2	30sec	2	30sec	2
1min	4	1min	4	1min	4
20sec	5	20sec	5	20sec	5
30sec	2	30sec	2	30sec	2
1min	4	1min	4	1min	4
20sec	5	20sec	5	20sec	5
2min	3	2min	3	2min	3
2min	2	2min	2	2min	2
1min	1	1min	1	1min	1

HOW HARD SHOULD YOU WORK?

Use this key to discover how much effort you should put in during every interval

1 Easy	2 Comfortable	3 Moderate	4 Intense	5 All-out

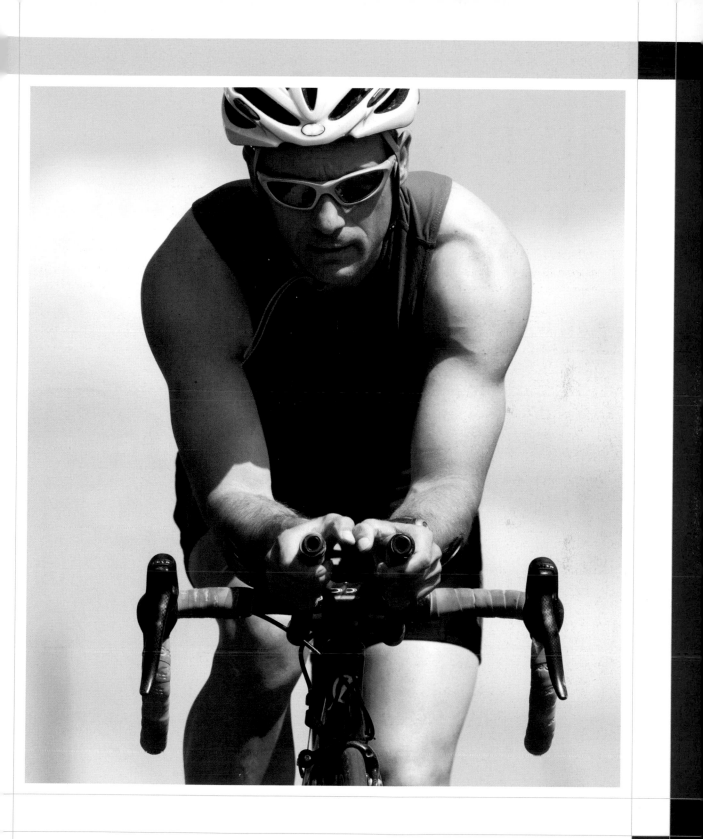

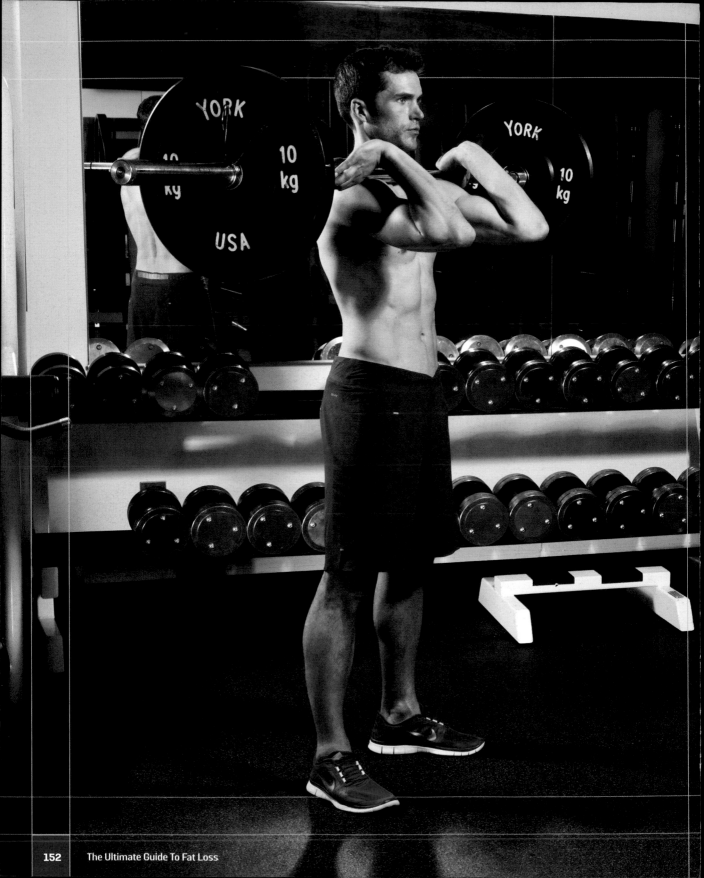

WEEK SIX

Turn the page for the **final week** of your
six-week nutrition and exercise plan

THIS WEEK'S MENU

MONDAY	TUESDAY	WEDNESDAY	THURSDAY

MONDAY

BREAKFAST
- Salmon fillet with 3 plum tomatoes and ½ avocado

SNACK
- Post-workout shake: blend 150ml coconut water, 1 scoop whey protein powder, 1 frozen banana, 1tbsp almond butter, 1tbsp ground flax seeds and ice

LUNCH
- 2 wholegrain wraps with Dijon mustard, sliced turkey breast, ½ avocado and goat's cheese

SNACK
- Chicken slices and almonds

DINNER
- Chicken wings with 40g brown rice, peas and chilli dipping sauce

SNACK
- Greek yoghurt with cinnamon

TUESDAY

BREAKFAST
- 2 poached eggs with roast beef slices

SNACK
- Greek yoghurt

LUNCH
- Chicken and vegetable skewers with a large green salad, drizzled with balsamic vinegar and olive oil

SNACK
- Hummus with carrot and pepper sticks

DINNER
- Cod fillet with asparagus and courgette

SNACK
- Banana and 30g whey protein shake

WEDNESDAY

BREAKFAST
- Salmon fillet with 3 plum tomatoes and ½ avocado

SNACK
- Post-workout shake: blend 150ml coconut water, 1 scoop whey protein powder, 1 frozen banana, 1tbsp almond butter, 1tbsp ground flax seeds and ice

LUNCH
- Salmon fillet with asparagus, peas and spinach, drizzled with 2tbsp extra virgin olive oil and lemon juice

SNACK
- 1 boiled egg chopped with mixed olives

DINNER
- Chicken breast with red pepper, cherry tomatoes, spinach, green beans and black olives, olive oil and balsamic vinegar

SNACK
- Greek yoghurt with cinnamon and almonds

THURSDAY

BREAKFAST
- Roast chicken slices and mixed vegetables

SNACK
- 1 slice toasted rye bread with cream cheese

LUNCH
- Ham and boiled egg salad

SNACK
- Greek yoghurt with cinnamon

DINNER
- Thai chicken curry with steamed mange tout and sugar snap peas

SNACK
- Bowl of blueberries and mixed nuts

Here's what you need to eat and when over the next seven days to blast away body fat

FRIDAY	SATURDAY	SUNDAY

FRIDAY

BREAKFAST
- Smoked salmon, 1 boiled egg and ½ avocado

SNACK
- Post-workout shake: blend 150ml coconut water, 1 scoop whey protein powder, 1 frozen banana, 1tbsp almond butter, 1tbsp ground flax seeds and ice

LUNCH
- 2 wholegrain wraps with Dijon mustard, sliced chicken breast, ½ avocado and goat's cheese

SNACK
- 1 apple and 12 almonds

DINNER
- Grilled ribeye steak with sweet potato mash, broccoli and a sprinkle of chilli flakes

SNACK
- Greek yoghurt with chopped banana

SATURDAY

BREAKFAST
- 2 poached eggs, 2 rashers grilled bacon and 2 grilled tomatoes

SNACK
- 50g reduced-fat cheese of your choice and 1 apple

LUNCH
- Ham and olive salad

SNACK
- 1 can tuna and spinach

DINNER
- Baked salmon with roasted vegetables

SNACK
- Natural yoghurt with blueberries, cinnamon and pecan nuts

SUNDAY

BREAKFAST
- 2 poached eggs, 2 rashers grilled bacon and 2 grilled tomatoes

SNACK
- Salsa with carrot and celery sticks

LUNCH
- Grilled chicken breast salad

SNACK
- 1 chopped boiled egg on 2 oatcakes

DINNER
- Seabass fillet with tomato salsa and broccoli florets

SNACK
- Greek yoghurt with mixed berries

SHAKE IT!
Protein shakes have been included on Monday, Wednesday and Friday because it's an effective way to plan your gym workouts. If you train on other days, have shakes after those sessions instead.

WORKOUTS

Congratulations! You've reached the final week of this six-week plan. By now you should have a well-established routine, which you should continue to follow. Don't be tempted to miss any workouts or fail to do the final high-intensity cardio session (see p170). All your efforts will be worth it.

WEEK SIX		EXERCISE	SETS	REPS	TEMPO	REST
WORKOUT 1	1A	Incline bench press	4	10	3010	10sec
	1B	Shoulder press	4	8	3010	10sec
	1C	Front raise	4	10	1010	10sec
	1D	Lateral raise	4	10	1010	120sec
	2A	Reverse-grip bent-over row	4	10	3010	10sec
	2B	Chin-up	4	8	3010	10sec
	2C	Cable reverse flye	4	10	2010	10sec
	2D	Cable straight-arm pull-down	4	10	2010	90sec

•• Perform the first sets of 1A, 1B, 1C and 1D, taking 10 seconds' rest between each. Then rest for 120 seconds and repeat until all four sets are completed.

•• Perform the first sets of 2A, 2B, 2C and 2D, taking 10 seconds' rest between each. Then rest for 90 seconds and repeat until all four sets are completed.

WEEK SIX — LOWER BODY

WORKOUT 2

	EXERCISE	SETS	REPS	TEMPO	REST
1A	Squat	4	10	2010	10sec
1B	Lunge	4	10	2010	10sec
1C	Calf raise	4	12	2110	10sec
1D	Box jump	4	10	X	120sec
2A	Hamstring curl	4	10	3010	10sec
2B	Leg press	4	12	2010	0sec
2C	Wide leg press	4	12	2010	0sec
2D	Narrow leg press	4	12	2010	120sec

•• Perform the first sets of 1A, 1B, 1C and 1D, taking 10 seconds' rest between each. Then rest for 120 seconds and repeat until all four sets are completed.

•• Perform the first set of 2A, rest for 10 seconds, then do the first sets of 2B, 2C and 2D without taking any rest between each. Then rest for 120 seconds and repeat until all four sets are completed.

WEEK SIX — TOTAL BODY

WORKOUT 3

	EXERCISE	SETS	REPS	TEMPO	REST
1A	Clean	4	10	X	10sec
1B	Push press	4	8	3010	10sec
1C	Romanian deadlift	4	10	2010	10sec
1D	Barbell shrug	4	10	1110	90sec
2A	Pull-up	4	6	3010	0sec
2B	Hanging leg raise	4	12	1110	0sec
2C	Hanging knee raise	4	12	1110	10sec
2D	Barbell rollout	4	8	3110	90sec

•• Perform the first sets of 1A, 1B, 1C and 1D, taking 10 seconds' rest between each. Then rest for 90 seconds and repeat until all four sets are completed.

•• Perform the first sets of 2A, 2B and 2C without taking any rest between each. Rest for 10 seconds, then do the first set of 2D. Rest for 90 seconds and repeat until all four sets are completed.

1A Incline bench press

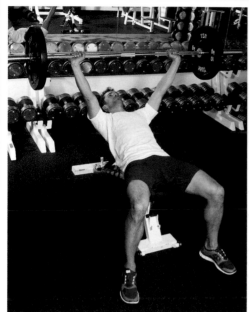
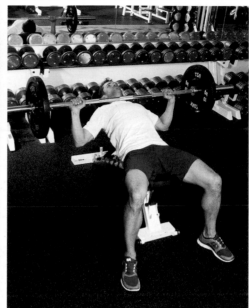

- Lie on a bench set at a 45° angle with your feet on the floor directly underneath your knees.
- Hold the bar with an overhand grip with your hands more than shoulder-width apart.
- Lower the bar towards your chest until your elbows are bent at 90° and the bar is almost touching the middle of your chest or is just above your nipples.
- Drive your feet hard into the floor and push the bar strongly back to the start.

1B Shoulder press

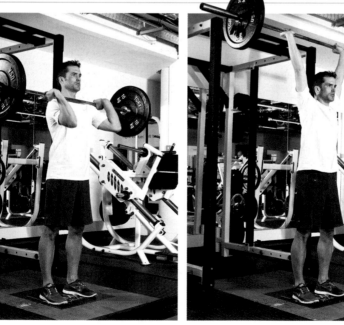

- Stand with your feet shoulder-width apart. Position a bar on your upper chest, gripping it with your hands slightly more than shoulder-width apart.
- Keep your chest upright and your core braced.
- Press the bar directly overhead until your arms are fully extended. Don't tilt your hips forwards.
- Lower the bar to return to the start.

1C Front raise

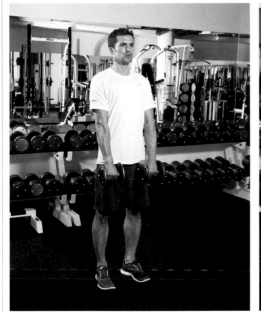 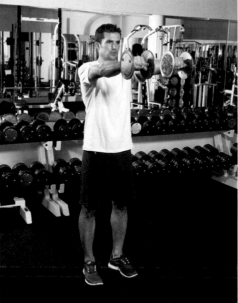

- Stand tall with your core braced and your feet shoulder-width apart, holding a light dumbbell in each hand in front of your thighs.
- Lift the weights in front of you, using your muscles and not momentum.
- Stop when the weights reach shoulder height. Lower to return to the start.

1D Lateral raise

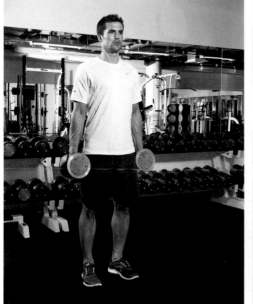 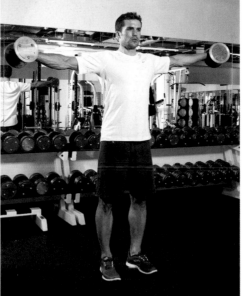

- Stand tall with your core braced and your feet shoulder-width apart, holding a light dumbbell in each hand by your sides with your palms facing your body.
- Leading with your elbows, lift the weights out to the sides, using your muscles and not momentum.
- Stop when the weights reach shoulder height. Lower to return to the start.

2A Reverse-grip bent-over row

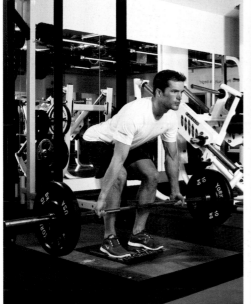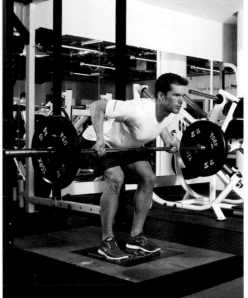

- Start with your core braced, your back straight and your shoulder blades retracted, gripping a bar with an underhand grip.
- Bend your knees slightly and lean forwards from the hips.
- Pull the bar up to your lower sternum, retracting your shoulder blades to allow the bar to come up to the chest, then lower again.

2B Chin-up

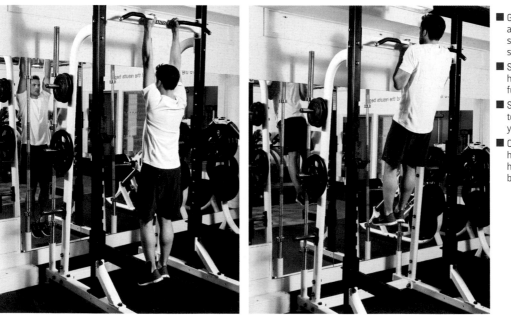

- Grab the bar with an underhand grip so your hands are shoulder-width apart.
- Start from a dead hang with your arms fully extended.
- Squeeze your lats together to pull yourself up.
- Once your chin is higher than your hands, lower yourself back to the start.

2C Cable reverse flye

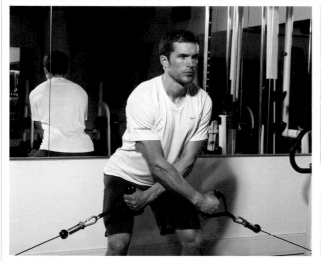
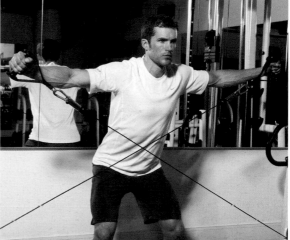

- Stand in the middle of a cable machine with your arms crossed, holding a D-handle attachment attached to the low pulley in each hand.
- Keeping your core braced and a slight bend in your elbows, lift both arms to shoulder height.
- Return to the start, maintaining control of the weight throughout.

2D Cable straight-arm pull-down

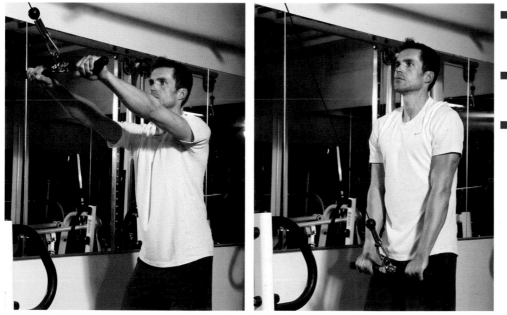

- Stand tall, holding a straight-bar handle attached to the high pulley of a cable machine.
- Keeping your arms straight, pull the bar down in an arc to your thighs.
- At the bottom of the move squeeze your lats and triceps and return to the start.

FAT-LOSS FINISHER
Burpee
p172

1A Squat

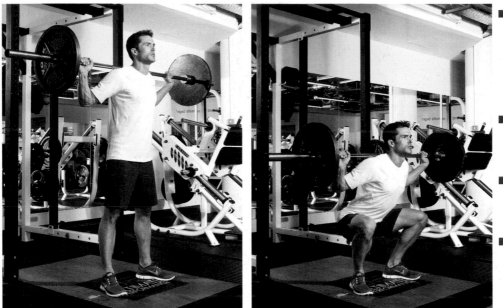

- Rest a barbell on the back of your shoulders – not your neck – holding it with an overhand grip slightly wider than your shoulders. Keep your elbows pointing to the floor.
- Your feet should be slightly more than shoulder-width apart with your toes pointing outwards slightly.
- Squat until your thighs are at least parallel to the floor, keeping your knees in line with your toes.
- Push back up through your heels to return to the start.

1B Lunge

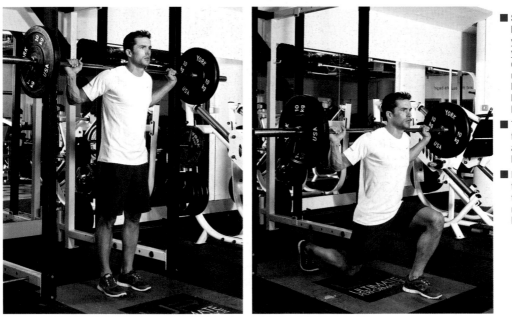

- Stand tall, resting a barbell on the back of your shoulders, not your neck. Point your elbows behind you to retract your shoulder blades, and keep your back upright and core braced throughout.
- Take a big step forwards with one leg and lunge until both knees are bent at 90°.
- Push back off your front foot to return to the start, then repeat with the other leg. That's one rep.

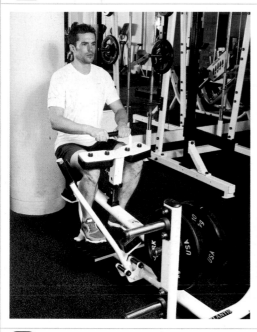
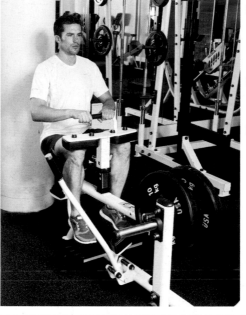

- Sit on the machine having adjusted the weight plates or stack, depending on the equipment, with your toes on the platform.
- Release the safety catch and go up on your tiptoes, keeping your body stable.
- Return to the start, making sure your heels go below the platform to achieve the full range of motion.

1D Box jump

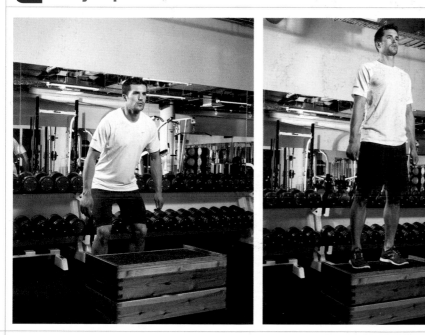

- Stand in front of a box or raised platform.
- Explosively jump on to the box, landing with both feet.
- Step back down to return to the start.

2A Hamstring curl

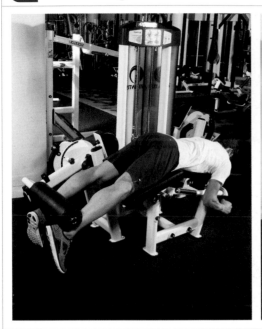
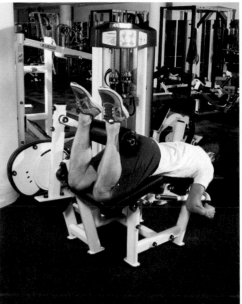

- Lie on your front on the machine, following the instructions to position yourself correctly and safely.
- With the pad against your lower calves, bend your knees and contract your hamstrings to raise it.
- Return to the start.

2B Leg press

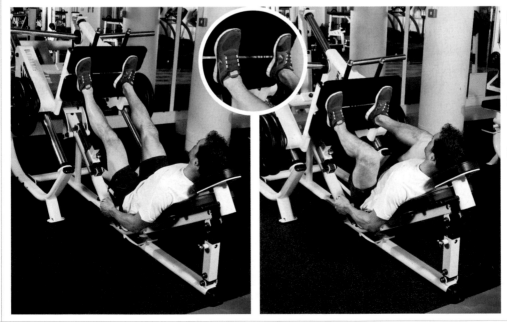

- Sit on the machine, following its instructions to position yourself correctly and safely, with your feet hip-width apart (see inset).
- Release the lock, bend your knees and slowly lower the platform towards you.
- Push through your heels to straighten your legs and return to the start.

2C Wide leg press

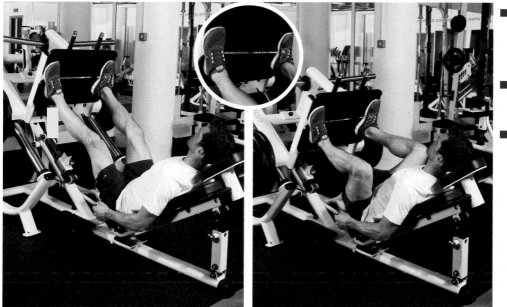

- Sit on the machine, following its instructions to position yourself correctly and safely, with your feet shoulder-width apart (see inset).
- Release the lock, bend your knees and slowly lower the platform towards you.
- Push through your heels to straighten your legs and return to the start.

2D Narrow leg press

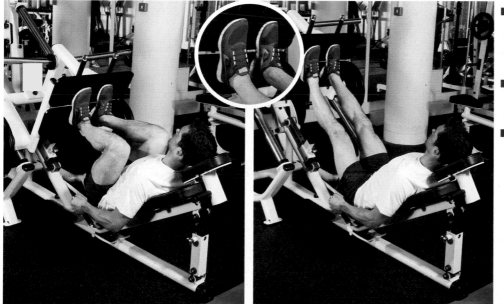

- Sit on the machine, following its instructions to position yourself correctly and safely, with your feet close together (see inset).
- Release the lock, bend your knees and slowly lower the platform towards you.
- Push through your heels to straighten your legs and return to the start.

FAT-LOSS FINISHER
Walking dumbbell lunge p177

1A Clean

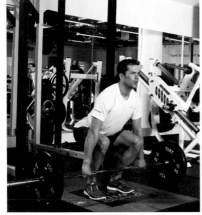 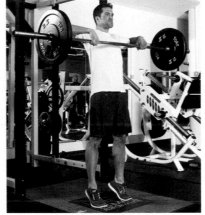 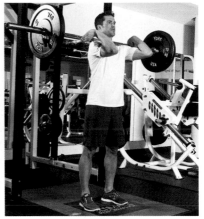

■ Stand with your feet shoulder-width apart so your shins are touching the bar. Squat and take hold of the bar with an overhand grip.

■ Keeping your core braced, your chest up and with a natural arch in your back, drive through your heels to lift the bar off the floor.

■ As the bar reaches your hips, rise on to your tiptoes, shrug your shoulders and pull the bar up higher, leading with your elbows.

■ As the bar travels towards your shoulders, squat under the bar and rotate your arms so your elbows face forwards

and you catch the bar on your fingers and the front of your shoulders.

■ Reverse the move to return to the start.

1B Push press

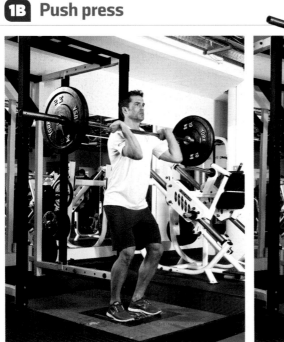 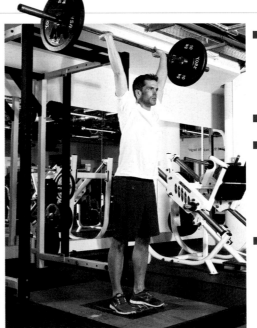

■ Stand with your feet shoulder-width apart. Position a bar on your upper chest, holding it so your hands are slightly more than shoulder-width apart.

■ Keep your chest upright and your core braced.

■ Bend at the knees to go into a quarter-squat, then stand up and press the bar directly overhead until your arms are fully extended. Don't tilt your hips forwards.

■ Lower the bar to return to the start.

1C Romanian deadlift

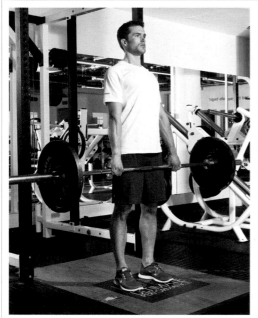
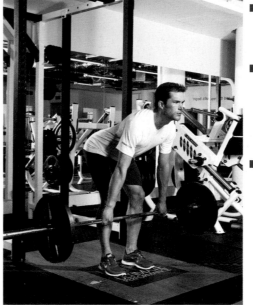

- Stand tall with your feet shoulder-width apart holding a barbell with an overhand grip just outside your thighs.
- Keeping a slight bend in your knees, lean forwards from your hips, not the waist, and lower the bar down the front of your shins until you feel a good stretch in your hamstrings.
- Reverse the move back to the start, pushing your hips forwards as you do so.

1D Barbell shrug

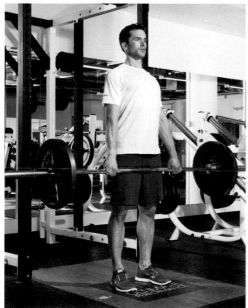
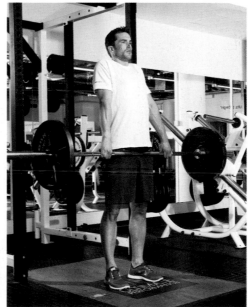

- Stand tall with your feet shoulder-width apart holding a barbell with an overhand grip just outside your thighs.
- Keeping your core braced and arms straight, shrug your shoulders towards your ears.
- Lower the weight back to the start.

2A Pull-up

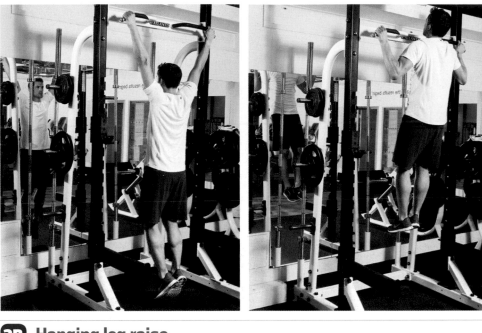

- Grab the bar with an overhand grip so your hands are more than shoulder-width apart.
- Start from a dead hang with your arms fully extended.
- Squeeze your lats together to pull yourself up.
- Once your chin is higher than your hands, lower yourself back to the start.

2B Hanging leg raise

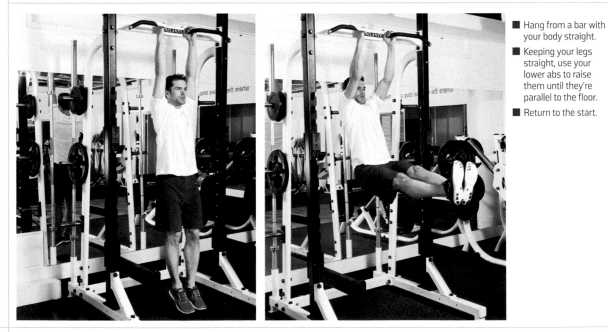

- Hang from a bar with your body straight.
- Keeping your legs straight, use your lower abs to raise them until they're parallel to the floor.
- Return to the start.

2C Hanging knee raise

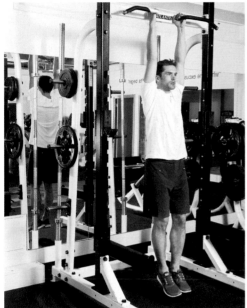 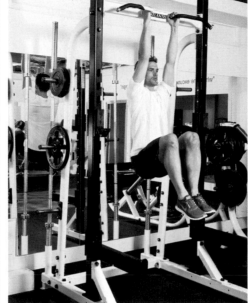

- Hang from a bar with your body straight.
- Bend your knees and use your lower abs to raise your legs until your thighs are parallel to the floor.
- Return to the start.

2D Barbell rollout

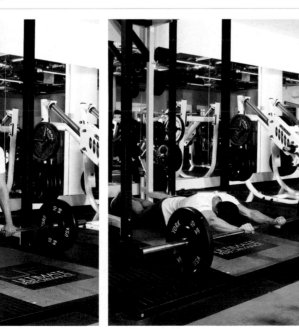

- Start on your knees with your arms extended and your hands holding a barbell with a shoulder-width grip.
- Roll the barbell away from your body, keeping your core braced.
- Once your torso is parallel to the floor, contract your abs and pull the bar back towards your body to return to the start.

FAT-LOSS FINISHER
Kettlebell swing
p173

GET MOVING

Choose your activity to complete this week's training programme

The fourth and final session of week six is a 25-minute high-intensity cardio session. Whether you run, cycle or row is up to you. To complete the session, simply follow the charts below to make sure you work your muscles and cardiovascular system to burn the optimum amount of body fat.

🏃 RUN		🚴 BIKE		🚣 ROW	
DURATION	**INTENSITY**	**DURATION**	**INTENSITY**	**DURATION**	**INTENSITY**
5min	2	5min	2	5min	2
5min	3	5min	3	5min	3
30sec	4	30sec	4	30sec	4
30sec	3	30sec	3	30sec	3
30sec	4	30sec	4	30sec	4
30sec	3	30sec	3	30sec	3
1min	4	1min	4	1min	4
30sec	3	30sec	3	30sec	3
1min	4	1min	4	1min	4
30sec	3	30sec	3	30sec	3
1min	4	1min	4	1min	4
20sec	5	20sec	5	20sec	5
30sec	2	30sec	2	30sec	2
1min	4	1min	4	1min	4
20sec	5	20sec	5	20sec	5
30sec	2	30sec	2	30sec	2
1min	4	1min	4	1min	4
20sec	5	20sec	5	20sec	5
2min	3	2min	3	2min	3
2min	2	2min	2	2min	2
1min	1	1min	1	1min	1

HOW HARD SHOULD YOU WORK?

Use this key to discover how much effort you should put in during every interval

1 Easy 2 Comfortable 3 Moderate 4 Intense 5 All-out

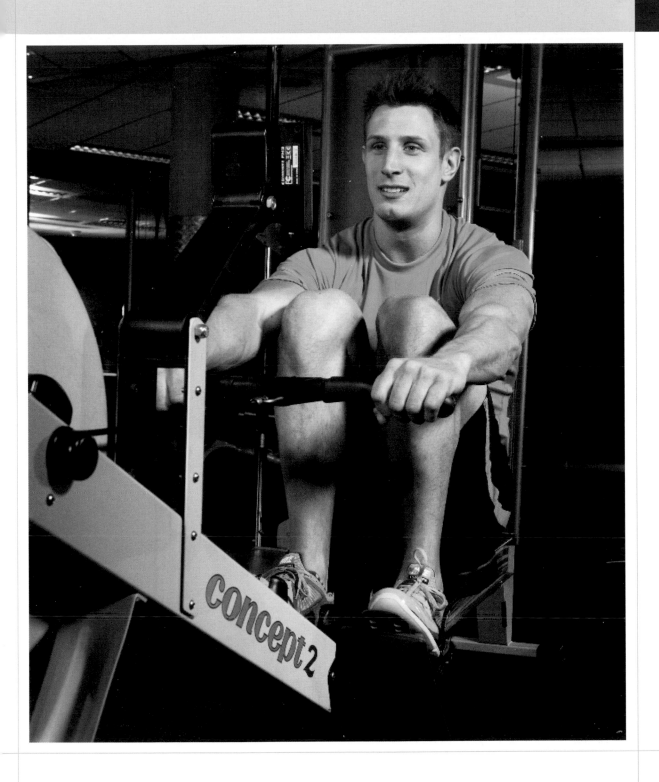

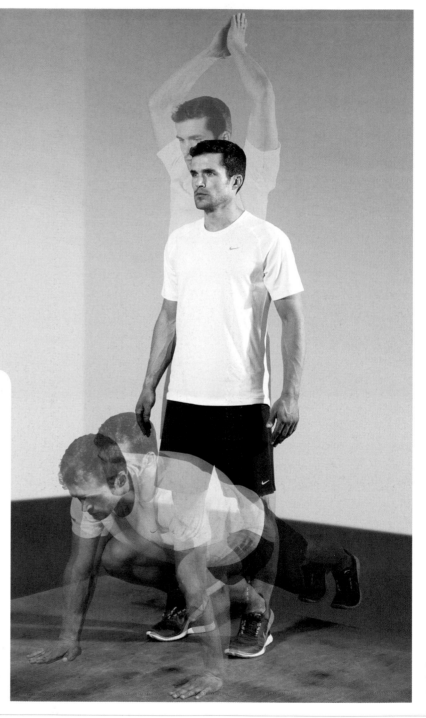

BURPEE
Sets 4 Reps 20
Rest 60sec

Why do it? This surprisingly tough bodyweight move hits all your major muscle groups and gets your heart and lungs working overtime to initiate a fat–burning response.

- Stand tall with your hands by your sides.
- Bend your knees and drop to the floor, placing your palms flat on the ground in front of you.
- Jump your legs out behind you so you're in a press-up position.
- Jump your knees back into your chest
- Jump up so your feet leave the floor. Land and go into the next rep.

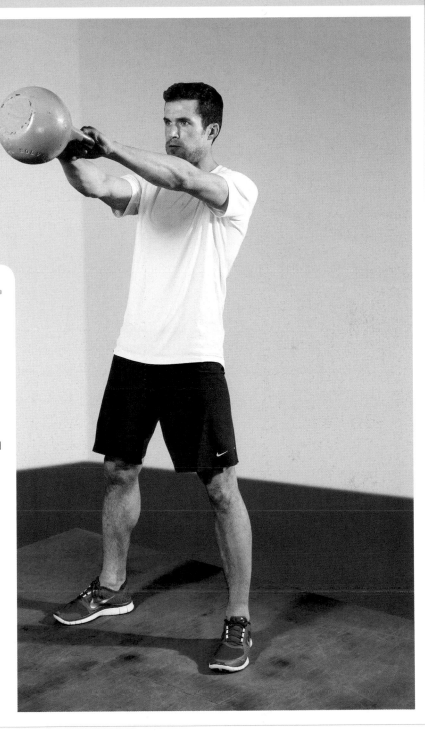

KETTLEBELL SWING

Sets 6 **Reps** 25
Rest 60sec

Why do it? This is one of
the best fat-stripping moves
because it gets your whole
body working as a single unit,
sends your heart rate soaring
and makes your abs work hard
to keep your torso stable.

- Stand with your feet shoulder-
  width apart, holding a kettlebell
  in front of you with both hands.

- Keeping your back straight and
  your knees in line with your feet,
  bend at the knees and move the
  kettlebell between your legs.

- Brace your core, stand up and
  snap your hips forwards to propel
  the kettlebell up to shoulder
  height. The power should come
  from your hips, not your arms.

- Breathe out at the top of the
  move and breathe in during
  the kettlebell's descent.

- Continue the swing in a fluid,
  controlled movement for the
  required number of reps.

FARMER'S WALK
Sets 8 Distance 25m Rest 60sec

Why do it? Walking while carrying additional weight works your cardiovascular system to create an oxygen debt and works your core to help build a six-pack.

- Stand in front of a long, clear pathway, holding a weighted bar or dumbbell in each hand.
- Keeping your core braced, walk as quickly as you can for the required distance.

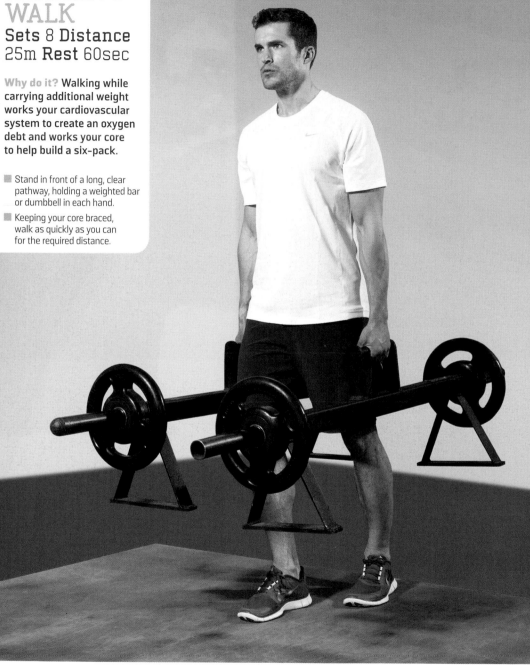

SPRINT
Sets 8 Distance
25m Rest 30sec

Why do it? Sprinting is one of the best ways to burn fat because the intense nature of the activity has the same effect on your body as weight training.

■ Stand in front of a long, clear pathway or on a treadmill.

■ Keeping your core braced and body upright, sprint the required distance.

SLED DRAG
Sets 8 Distance 25m Rest 30sec

Why do it? The additional weight and drag of the sled means you have to give it everything to get it moving, which works your heart and lungs, plus all your major muscle groups.

- Stand with your back to a long, clear pathway, holding a sled strap in each hand.
- Keeping your core braced and your arms straight, drag the sled along the path for the required distance.

WALKING DUMBBELL LUNGE

Sets 4 Distance 25m Rest 30sec

Why do it? Not only will this move work your quads, hams, glutes and abs, it will also get your heart and lungs out of their comfort zone so you get fitter and leaner.

- Stand in front of a long, clear pathway, holding a dumbbell in each hand.
- Keeping your core braced, take a big step forwards and lunge until both knees are bent at 90°.
- Push off from your back foot and lunge forwards with that leg.
- Repeat until you've covered the required distance.